STANDARDIZING BIOMECHANICAL TESTING IN SPORT

David A. Dainty
Canadian Memorial Chiropractic College

Robert W. Norman
University of Waterloo

Human Kinetics Publishers, Inc.
Champaign, IL

Library of Congress Cataloging-in-Publication Data

Dainty, David A., 1946–
  Standardizing biomechanical testing in sport.

  Bibliography: p.
  Includes index.
  1. Sports—Physiological aspects. 2. Human mechanics.
3. Athletic ability. I. Norman, Robert W., 1941–
II. Title. [DNLM: 1. Biomechanics. 2. Kinetics.
3. Movement. 4. Sports. WE 103 D133s]
RC1235.D35 1987   612'.044   86-15391
ISBN 0-87322-074-9

Senior Editor: Sue Wilmoth, PhD
Production Director: Ernie Noa
Assistant Production Director: Lezli Harris
Copy Editor: Ann Breuhler
Proofreader: Lise Rodgers
Typesetter: Brad Colson
Text Layout: Lezli Harris
Cover Design: Jack Davis
Printed by: Braun-Brumfield, Inc.

ISBN: 0-87322-074-9

Printed in the United States of America

10 9 8 7 6 5 4 3 2 1

Human Kinetics Publishers, Inc.
Box 5076, Champaign, IL   61820

Contents

Contributors   v

Preface   vii

Acknowledgments   ix

1: Biomechanical Testing Procedures   1

Defining a Problem   2
Units of Measure   2
Definitions   3
Ethics and Safety   3
Detailed Reporting   4
Data Bases   4
Frequency of Testing   4
Innovative Techniques   5
Strategies for Research   5
Conclusion and Recommendations   8

2: Kinematics   9

Purpose for Measuring   11
Relevance   11
Testing Procedures   11
Interpretation of Test Results   19
Kinematic Written Reports   20

3: Kinetics   21

Physical Properties of the Limbs and Total Body   21
Forces, Impulse, and Momentum   31
Mechanical Energy, Work, and Efficiency   46

4: Neuromuscular Considerations   59

Definition and Explanation of the Parameters   60
Purpose for Measuring the Different Neuromuscular   62
  Parameters and Their Relevance
Testing Procedures   64
Interpretation of Test Results   67

5: Recommended Procedures   73

Cinematography   74
Sampling Rate and Data Smoothing   80
Direct Measurement Techniques   81
Physical Properties of the Limbs and the Total Body   83
Muscular Forces and Moments and Joint Reaction Forces 84
Force and Pressure Transducers   85
Impulses and Momenta   91
Neuromuscular Measurement (EMG)   98
Summary   100

Appendix A: International System of Units (SI)   101

Appendix B: Policy Statement Regarding the Use   105
of Human Subjects and Informed Consent

Appendix C: Units, Terms, and Standards in the   109
Reporting of EMG Research

Appendix D: Sample Budget   131

References   133

Index   145

About the Contributors

David A. Dainty is the Academic Dean of the Canadian Memorial Chiropractic College in Toronto, Ontario. Professor Micheline Gagnon teaches biomechanics in the Department of Physical Education at the University of Montréal. Pierre Lagasse is an associate professor in the Department of Physical Education at Laval University in Ste-Foy, Quebec. Robert Norman is a professor of biomechanics in the Department of Kinesiology at the University of Waterloo. Gordon Robertson is an assistant professor of biomechanics at the University of Ottawa. Eric Sprigings is an associate professor of biomechanics in the college of Physical Education at the University of Saskatchewan in Saskatoon.

Preface

Six individuals with a strong commitment to biomechanics and sport were selected to write this text on testing elite athletes by using biomechanical analyses. This book is a continuation of the Sport Canada program to standardize testing in the physiological and psychomotor areas.

Unlike other biomechanics texts that exclusively address either theory or techniques, we have blended these two areas. While providing some basic theory, we intentionally approached the theoretical part in terms of application to testing. The text is comprised of five chapters that effectively divide the subject matter into divisions related to the type of testing one would typically use in a sport situation.

The first four chapters are devoted to an explanation of the underlying principles concerned with kinematics, kinetics, work-energy, body segment parameters, and the neuromuscular basis of human movement. These chapters are well documented and explain the premises on which the techniques in chapter 5 are based. Chapter 5 is devoted entirely to the techniques that are used in the biomechanical evaluation of elite athletes. Although many techniques are discussed, they are by no means all-inclusive; other tests or variations of the ones discussed may be just as applicable under certain situations. This approach also leaves room for innovation in developing new tests. Appendix A is a compilation of the international system of units. Appendix B gives the American College of Sports Medicine's policy statement on using human research subjects. The International Society of Electrophysiology Kinesiology's units, terms, and standards used in reporting EMG research comprise Appendix C. New researchers will appreciate the sample budget for a filming project presented in Appendix D.

The book was written for researchers at Canadian universities who are actively evaluating elite athletes. The text should also serve as a reference book for undergraduate and graduate students in biomechanics of sport and for coaches, technical directors, and sport administrators who make fiscal decisions concerning testing and evaluation programs for their athletes.

David A. Dainty
Robert W. Norman

Acknowledgments

As with any text, the authors are not the only contributors to the completion of the manuscript. We would especially like to thank Mrs. Joan Pache of the University of Waterloo Department of Kinesiology for the typing and proofreading of the manuscript and for many constructive comments about the style and wording of several sections. The contributions of colleagues and students from all institutions are also greatly appreciated. Finally, the support and understanding of the Canadian Association of Sport Sciences and the Canadian Society for Biomechanics must be recognized, for without them the realization of this publication would have been impossible.

1

Biomechanical Testing Procedures

DAVID DAINTY
MICHELINE GAGNON

Standardizing testing procedures in biomechanics of sport research is a difficult task. Because the data collection process in biomechanics is so highly dependent on technological advances, the rapid changes that have occurred and are still taking place preclude definitive techniques being described. These changes have come about in hardware, software, and applications. For example, the development of the electrogoniometer from a quite simple measuring device to one that allows for nonplanar movement has changed the data base for joint angle studies. The development of rigorous data processing and analysis procedures (spline functions, Fourier analysis, and digital filters) has changed the whole concept of what to believe in interpreting both collected raw data and mathematically derived data. Finally, the continual advancements in the field of microelectronics, or high technology, are providing us daily with new instrumentation and techniques to give more and better information on such subjects as pressure distribution under the foot and tendon and ligament tension in vivo.

The preceding examples are but a few of the vast changes taking place; consequently, the task of saying what is correct and what is not, in terms of techniques, is very difficult. However, some fundamental laws, principles, and procedures must be followed in biomechanics testing as in any discipline.

The word biomechanics has very broad implications in many areas of research and, as with other sciences, does not stand alone in its application. Many exercise physiologists are looking at certain phenomena in muscle that are quite mechanical in nature. Many biomechanists are also

1

studying problems that have physiological implications such as energy systems and the relationships between internal and external work and efficiency. To isolate the area of biomechanics and more specifically, sport biomechanics, would be unjustified and incorrect. Consequently, many techniques and standardized processes from other disciplines apply equally to biomechanics.

Defining a Problem

In examining any sport or any measurable phenomenon, one must be aware of the limitations, procedures, and most importantly, the goals of the work to be performed. In answering questions concerning these goals, it is important to differentiate the problem as either a research or a testing situation. Is the work performed designed to answer basic questions and advance the knowledge in the area, or is it simply a test situation to define how athletes compare to one another or to some normative data? Sometimes the problem is somewhat unclear and a number of prerequisites must be established prior to beginning a project. The first of these prerequisites is a clear statement of the problem. This statement will come from an understanding of not only what is required but what has happened in the past by exhaustively reviewing related literature, sorting out much of the misinformation, and proposing an explanation of what is to be done.

In preparing these preliminary documents, the researcher needs to differentiate the problem into a qualitative or quantitative study. The qualitative study handles descriptive information and may or may not include measurement, whereas the quantitative study is more rigorous in both the experimental setup and the design. Both of these types of studies have a place in sport investigation, but the researcher must be aware of the nature of the questions being asked to adequately use either form.

Units of Measure

In defining any type of study, certain standards and norms must be followed so that basic information can be obtained and communicated. The most basic norms are those involving units of measurement. The language of science in this area is the Système International (SI) or, as it is more commonly called, the metric system. The units of measure in this system are such units as meters (length), kilograms (mass), Newtons (force), and watts (power). A more exhaustive list is contained in Appendix A, including multiplication factors and prefixes. When using these values in an experimental report the investigator should consider the audience and its comprehension of SI. Although most countries of the world accept and use SI, one notable exception is the United States. Scientists throughout the world, however, use this system in their communications.

Definitions

Many definitions in biomechanics literature and jargon sometimes present difficulty. The confusion arises because of the seeming similarity between terms or the relative unfamiliarity with certain terms by researchers. In the former category are such terms as joint reaction forces and bone-on-bone forces. Joint reaction forces plus the active muscular forces create the bone-on-bone forces (Winter, 1979a) and care must be taken in describing and analyzing forces that occur about a joint. In the latter category are many terms that may be indigenous to a particular study or discipline, but are not commonly found in the literature. To give a list of these would be difficult and likely not all-inclusive. Therefore, during the course of the next three chapters, definitions peculiar to certain tests shall be presented. In any particular study, the researcher should define terms that may be ambiguous or misunderstood.

Ethics and Safety

In performing any tests that require the use of human subjects, care must be taken to ensure their safety and well-being. In most Canadian universities, an ethics committee reviews all research proposals involving human subjects. This practice ensures that an objective evaluation of experimental procedures is performed and that ethical norms are followed. To this end, several agencies such as the Canada Council and the Medical Research Council have published guidelines on ethical procedures in research involving human subjects. The American College of Sports Medicine has also published a policy statement on the use of human subjects which is contained in Appendix B.

One of the more important aspects of ensuring the subjects' safety is to inform them of the risks, hazards, and nature of the testing to be performed and to receive their written permission to perform such tests. This type of permission form is mandatory for most ethical reviews and should include a description of the test with possible dangers. Also included in this form should be a place for the signatures of the subject and a witness to demonstrate that the subject is fully aware of all procedures.

Detailed Reporting

As was mentioned in a preceding section, a difference exists between a qualitative and quantitative type of study and also between studies involving testing only and those that are research-oriented. Many testing-type studies are required for sport governing bodies. These studies involve little in the way of any research information. However, the same rigorous pursuit of excellence is needed as would be found in a research project. Although the experimental and research design will not be included in a testing situation, the same detail in testing and concern for the subjects and resulting data should exist. Also, the validity and reliability of any test or evaluation procedure should be identified so that interpretation of the results provides useful and meaningful information. To treat a testing or evaluation project as less rigorous or less important than a research project is doing the testing project a disservice. Downplaying this attention to detail leads to much misinformation in the literature and causes conflicts when similar studies are attempted.

Data Bases

An important aspect of research that has not received much attention in biomechanics studies is the development of broad data bases. Because of changes in technology, the relative newness of the science, and the development of techniques and procedures, many studies in the literature have involved small groups of subjects or solely methodology. The need to expand our subject populations and so increase our data base is of great importance. This need is another reason why particular attention must be paid to experimental design, testing protocol, and subject safety, so that studies can be replicated and the amount of data on certain parameters can be greatly expanded. The expansion of data bases and sample populations will enhance the use and interpretation of statistical methods in biomechanical studies.

Frequency of Testing

Coincidentally, with expanding data bases, a need exists for developing repeated testing bouts on the same group of subjects. Care must be taken in repeated tests to ensure that the parameter being investigated is not influenced by outside sources. For instance, if the effect of strength training on a particular skill is being investigated, the consequence of learning the skill must be accounted for by using, perhaps, a nontrained group. Although this is a simple example, the point of isolating the parameters under investigation is necessary. A realization of the confounding influences must also be documented.

In a sport setting, the frequency of testing should be determined in consultation with the coach and athlete to find when the evaluation process will be most beneficial. Some testing that requires the subject to change his or her normal movement patterns through the introduction of equipment or invasive techniques should be avoided just prior to a competition. However, nonrestrictive testing involving filming, force platforms, or other nonlimiting protocols may be quite useful before competition for the evaluation of technique. The decision and the design of protocol for frequency of testing must also be carefully considered. Although a need exists for larger data bases and increased testing frequency to establish repeatability and reliability, these should not be included to the disadvantage of the athlete.

Innovative Techniques

Although many examples of tests and testing protocols are described and suggested in the ensuing chapters, they are by no means the only tests that can be used. A certain amount of leeway must be available for the development of new protocols and the advancement of techniques. This manual is not intended to be restrictive in terms of stifling ingenuity. The intent is to provide guidelines to those who are testing athletes. The development of new, creative methods for the evaluation of certain parameters must also be recognized as part of the overall process of athlete testing. It is hoped that many of the suggestions in the following chapters will be implemented in any investigation involving athletes. However, the suggestions are not meant to be so restrictive as to prevent innovation and creativity.

Strategies for Research

The development and use of any test protocol requires a certain strategy to be followed to obtain a desired result. The establishment of research strategies for the analysis of the biomechanical aspects of sport motion is discussed here. Included are some basic definitions and points of information. The suggestions contained in this section will be further expanded in later chapters.

Any problem-solving is based on a *scientific theory* that includes some statements related to a body of knowledge. The theory is designed to fulfill a descriptive, explicative, and prognostic function. For instance, the theory of elasticity is the body of knowledge that involves the distribution of stress and strain in various elastic bodies subjected to given loads, displacements, and distributions of temperature. A *method* is a system of rules or principles that guides the experimental analyses. For example, with the theory of elasticity, the method of finite elements could be used to predict stress distributions on the spine when it is submitted to specific loads. A *procedure* is a generalized way of tackling a particular kind of analysis and may involve a set of techniques. For instance, the stress distribution on the spine could be analyzed through procedures of mathematical modeling. A *technique* is a specific way of acquiring evidence. In the preceding problem, tridimensional techniques could be combined with strain gauge measurements of the spine in vitro to collect the pertinent data.

A problem analysis must be very broad in the way that all the information pertaining to its comprehension is identified. The first step consists of establishing the purpose. The main goals generally sought in biomechanical analysis of sport are the following:

1. To provide *diagnostic tools* for the evaluation of performance and the evaluation of trauma associated with sport activities.
2. To provide *recommendations* concerning the factors related to *performance and safety* (relations between man—motion—environment).
3. To provide *recommendations* concerning the *training* and *teaching methods* for improving performance and recommendations to evaluate *therapeutic methods* used in the treatment of sport injuries.

To fulfill this problem analysis strategy, the next three chapters are designed in the following manner:

- Introduction
- Purpose for Measuring
- Relevance
- Testing Procedures
- Interpretation of Test Results
- Other Material

Using these subheadings will help the researcher or test group to establish relevant problems and undertake acceptable protocols to answer the questions demanded by the problems identified.

The use of problem and task analysis is quite helpful in organizing a research or testing project. Before beginning to utilize the methods, procedures, and techniques established for answering the specific questions asked, certain background material is imperative.

First the researcher must establish those factors associated with a given task in order to identify the performance or the risk elements in sport by examining the interaction between the individual, his or her task (sport activity), and the environment.

- *Characteristics of population*: age, sex, morphology, level of training, level of expertise, and so on.
- *Motion analysis*: motion patterns (spatiotemporal, external forces generated at the points of supports, and internal forces exerted on the bony structures) through kinematic and kinetic analyses; distinctions between different techniques (based on different velocities, loads or motion patterns); distinctions between normal and abnormal states (fatigue effects, traumatisms, etc.).
- *Environmental analysis*: sport equipment, floor surfaces, walls, and so on.
- *Interactions* among the preceding factors.

These preliminary analyses are based on a comprehensive and extensive review of the literature. At this point, the researcher should be able to identify some of the factors that appear to have some effect on performance or sport injuries for a global understanding of the problem.

Next the researcher can proceed to the specific measuring protocols that will lead to a solution of the problem. Table 1 outlines the various

Table 1.1 Biomechanical Parameters and Techniques

Subject Area	Parameters	Techniques
Physical properties of segments	Joint centers, masses, centers of mass, moments of inertia	Norms, regression equations, models, direct measurement
Kinematics	Time, displacement, velocity acceleration, strain	Timers, measurement devices, filming (planar and tridimensional), electrogoniometers (planar and 3-D), accelerometers, potentiometers, photooptical devices, computer simulation, and so on
Kinetics	Forces, impulses, pressure distribution, stress	Pressure transducers, force transducers (piezoelectric, piezoresistive, ceramic, strain gauge), force platforms, filming (planar, 3-D) modeling, EMG
Electrical and electromechanical properties	Thresholds, MVC, contractile properties, muscle structure, activation, sequencing	EMG, anatomical techniques (dissection, electronmicroscope, and so on)

parameters of interest in biomechanical investigation and some of the techniques used to examine them. The following four chapters are dedicated to detailing these parameters.

Conclusion and Recommendations

Our type of approach suggested for solving biomechanical problems requires the formation of a multidisciplinary research team including sport biomechanists, mechanical and biomedical engineers, and physicians. Isolated research should not be discouraged, but substantial progress toward the understanding of a given problem with its multidimensional aspects can be more easily achieved through a multidisciplinary research team. The different fields of knowledge should be integrated by clearly defining the common research strategies required to approach the problem. This integration implies an extensive collaboration among the team members.

A global understanding of the problem should be based on careful examinations of the sport situations and on the identification of the factors affecting the performance or the factors that could be associated with sport injuries. The research tools should be examined, redesigned, or redefined according to their appropriateness for the problem investigated, and the preceding information combined with the information regarding the modeling procedures should be used to develop a model. This model should serve as a tool in predicting the performance and safety factors involved in the sport situations and in evaluating the training methods and the therapeutic treatments of sport injuries.

The use of biomechanical testing procedures is not a simple or straightforward task. The implementation and interpretation of the same test procedures may be quite diverse among investigators. The next chapters are an attempt to overcome these discrepancies for sport evaluation and allow for the development of more rigid protocols.

2

Kinematics

GORDON ROBERTSON
ERIC SPRIGINGS

Kinematics is the branch of mechanics that is concerned with the description of how a body moves in space. Kinematics does not try to explain the cause behind the observed motion.

The following kinematic parameters can be measured:

1. Time[1]
2. Position
3. Linear displacement
4. Linear velocity
5. Linear acceleration
6. Angular displacement
7. Angular velocity
8. Angular acceleration

Table 2.1 lists acceptable units of measurement for kinematic data.

Kinematic parameters must be measured accurately if they are going to reflect the true movement history of a body. The accuracy of measured kinematic parameters is especially important if these parameters are to serve as input to subsequent kinetic analyses or model validation. In general, kinematic parameter values that arise from measurements taken on the observed motion of an actual physical point will be reasonably accurate, provided that the researcher adheres to proper protocol. On the other hand, kinematic measurements on derived mathematical points

[1]Strictly speaking, time is not considered to be a kinematic parameter. It is generally considered under a separate heading called *temporal analysis*.

Table 2.1 Units of Measurement for Kinematic Data

Kinematic Parameter	Abbreviation	SI Unit
Time	t	second
Position		
Rectangular coordinates		
(2-D or 3-D)	x, y, (z)	meter, meter, meter
Polar (2-D)	r, θ	meter, radian
Cylindrical (3-D)	r, θ, z	meter, radian, meter
Spherical (3-D)	ϱ, θ, ϕ	meter, radian, radian
Linear displacement	s	meter (m)
Linear velocity	ν	meters per second (m/s)
Linear acceleration	a	meters per second per second (m/s^2)
Angular displacement	θ	radian (rad)
Angular velocity	ω	radians per second (rad/s)
Angular acceleration	α	radians per second per second (rad/s^2)

such as the center of gravity (CG) of a segment(s) will prove to be less reliable as a result of the uncertainty about how well the derived point reflects the motion of the intended point.

Acceleration (angular, linear) is, perhaps, the most difficult of the kinematic parameters to measure accurately. Acceleration values derived from the displacement history of a body are meaningless unless proper techniques have been employed prior to differentiation. The major problems arise from nonsystematic errors found in the raw data, and are identified as noise. For a more in-depth discussion on acceptable smoothing techniques, the reader is referred to the section, Sampling Rate and Data Smoothing, in chapter 5.

Angular measurements between segments of the human body are quite often difficult to obtain accurately. The main reason for this difficulty is that the instantaneous joint center is often hard to identify. The hip, shoulder, and knee joints provide examples of this situation. Angular measurements that involve the trunk are notoriously difficult to accurately measure as a result of the additional complexities posed by a nonrigid segment.

Purpose for Measuring

Kinematic parameters are mere descriptors of an observed motion. They offer no explanation as to how or why an event took place. Thus they should be thought of as a starting place for an analysis rather than an end result. The main value derived from measuring kinematic parameters is that they serve as the basic input from which all subsequent kinetic calculations will be made. The reliability (i.e., accuracy and precision) of any kinetic measurement can only be as good as the reliability of the underlying kinematic data. Thus accuracy must be achieved in the measurement of any kinematic parameter. The accurate measurement of kinematic parameters is of fundamental importance in the evaluation of sport performances because it is these kinematic parameters that form the building blocks from which many subsequent kinetic calculations may be made.

Relevance

Few would argue with the statement that kinematic motion analyses have proven useful in the early conceptual stages of understanding a given sport technique. However, most sports have now progressed to the point where mere description is not adequate. What is required is a deeper understanding of the underlying reasons (i.e., kinetic analyses) that make a certain technique superior to that of another.

Undoubtedly, such kinematic display techniques as angle-angle diagrams and time-history graphs of displacement, velocity, and acceleration have proven their worth in allowing comparisons to be made between athletic performances. These comparisons can either be between the repeated performances of the same subject or between the performances of different subjects. But as was mentioned previously, the shortcoming of solely relying on the kinematic approach is that it fails to probe into the reasons behind the observed differences. The measurement of kinematic parameters is appropriate for all sports, but these measurements should *not* be thought of as the final end product.

Testing Procedures

The following is a list of the more commonly used kinematic measurement techniques. A brief statement is also added with regard to the inherent strengths and weaknesses of each of the techniques. A more detailed discussion on the specific testing protocol required for each of the measurement techniques may be found in chapter 5.

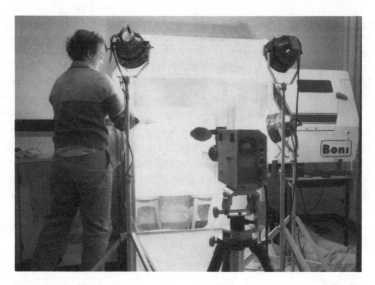

Figure 2.1   Typical 16mm camera.

CINEMATOGRAPHY

This method of measurement employs the use of motion picture cameras in the gathering of the kinematic parameters. The 16mm movie camera (see Figure 2.1) has been the common choice of most researchers because it offers a compromise between qualitative accuracy and expense. However, super 8mm cameras have recently become more viable due to the availability of higher speed super 8 cameras and the supporting super 8 film analyzers. In the final analysis, it will be the nature (precision and frequency domain) of the data that will dictate the type of movie camera that should be employed.

Advantages.

- One of the major advantages of the cinematographical approach is the flexibility that it provides in the research setting. For example, the researcher is permitted the choice of either a two-dimensional or three-dimensional investigation depending, of course, on the nature of the problem. The subject's normal movement pattern is not hampered by the attachment of external measuring devices.
- The accuracy of the cinematographical approach can be good if the appropriate filming and analytical protocol is followed.

Disadvantages.

- The major disadvantage of the cinematographical approach to date has been the rather lengthy delay that exists between the actual

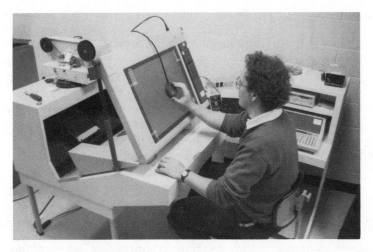

Figure 2.2 Computer linked film digitizer.

filming stage and the final results. This extended turn-around time is due to film processing, data reduction by digitizing, and other means (see Figure 2.2).

SINGLE-PLATE METHODS

Four kinematic measurement techniques fall under this general classification. The four techniques are

1. stroboscopy,
2. rotating-slit shutter,
3. light-streak photography, and
4. interrupted-light photography.

The common bond among these four techniques is that they all attempt to record the sequence of motion on a single frame of film. The general method for all four techniques is to leave the shutter open on a camera and then regulate the amount of admitted light to the film by various means.

The following are a few of the advantages and disadvantages provided by this classification of measurement technique.

Advantages.

- The setup is relatively simple and inexpensive.
- Analyses can begin almost immediately if a Polaroid-type camera is used.

Disadvantages.

- The overlapping of images often obscures the sought-after landmarks on a given body.
- These techniques are generally limited to two-dimensional displacement data.
- Generally, the subject will have to perform in subdued lighting, which could prove hazardous as well as produce unrepresentative data for the sought-after movement pattern.
- If stroboscopy is used, the flickering strobe light may upset a subject's normal movement pattern. In fact, movements that require accurate visual feedback by the subject may prove to be too difficult.

OPTOELECTRIC MOVEMENT MONITORING SYSTEM

These types of systems are generally comprised of light-emitter(s) attached to the point of interest on the body (see Figure 2.3), a remote receiver (see Figure 2.4), and some sort of microprocessing system

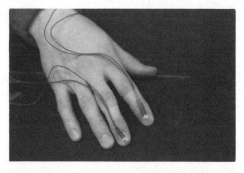

Figure 2.3 Light emitting diodes on subject.

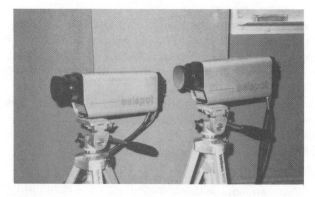

Figure 2.4 "Selspot" light receiving camera.

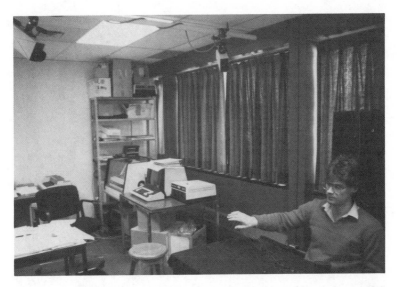

Figure 2.5 Experimental set-up using "Watsmart" optoelectric monitoring system (note cameras near ceiling).

designed to compute the displacement function of the body (see Figure 2.5). Additional software can be written to compute the higher order derivatives of the displacement function.

Advantage.

- These types of systems permit instantaneous analyses.

Disadvantages.

- As a result of the emitters being attached directly to the surface of the body, any movement of the soft tissue covering the actual skeletal landmark of interest will seriously reduce the accuracy of the measurement.
- As with any measurement system that comes in direct contact with the subject, the question is raised concerning the degree of hindrance it provides to the subject's normal movement pattern.

TELEVISION SYSTEMS

Generally, this type of measurement system has a fixed scanning rate that permits a maximum sampling rate of 60 Hertz (Hz). This sampling rate of 60 Hz is suitable for most gross human movement studies but would certainly be inadequate in quantitative analyses involving, for example, human impact phenomena (Figure 2.6).

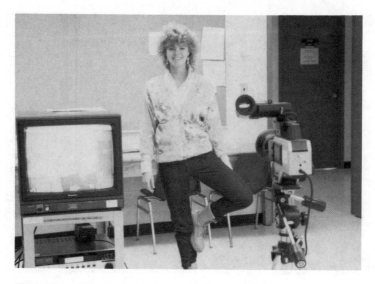

Figure 2.6 TV camera and monitoring system.

Advantage.

• This method provides the possibility of an instant replay for an initial qualitative assessment. The time and expense required for processing of film also is eliminated.

Disadvantages.

• This method provides a relatively low maximum sampling rate.
• Image resolution is inferior to that of, for instance, 16mm movie film.

ACCELEROMETERS

As the name suggests, accelerometers are devices that directly measure acceleration (Figure 2.7). They can be used singly or in groups of two, three (triaxial), five, six, or even nine, if greater accuracy is required. When the complete spatial (i.e., three-dimensional) motion of a body segment is required, six properly oriented accelerometers are needed, although Morris (1973) used only five and Padgaonkar, Krieger, and King (1975) recommended nine. Single accelerometers are used when only linear motion is to be studied (Bishop, 1976), whereas simple rotatory motions require two accelerometers (e.g., Pezzack, Norman, & Winter, 1977).

Triaxial accelerometers may be purchased that contain three premounted accelerometers all perpendicular to one another (see Figure 2.7). These devices are often used for head impact research (Bishop, 1977;

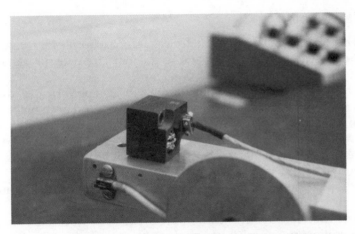

Figure 2.7 Triaxial (top) and uniaxial (side) accelerometers mounted on device for measuring arm accelerations.

Gersten, Orr, Sexton, & Okin, 1969; Norman, Bishop, Pierrynowski, & Pezzack, 1979). When used in total body motion studies, the results can be interpreted only as estimates of the total body motion because the human body is not well represented as a point mass (Winter, 1979b).

Accelerometers can be of piezoelectric, piezoresistive, or strain-gauge design. The selection of a particular design will depend upon the specific application. The piezoelectric (Bishop, 1976) models are the most common commercially but, unfortunately, suffer from having no steady-state response and may not be appropriate for slow or stationary human mechanics research. The piezoresistive (Norman, Bishop et al., 1979) and strain-gauge (Morris, 1973) designs do have steady-state responses but can be easily damaged if inadvertently dropped or struck by a hard material.

The most common and appropriate use of accelerometers is to measure acceleration when they are mounted on rigid materials. These materials may be mechanical models or parts of the human body (e.g., anthropomorphic dummies or head forms).

Advantages.

- The devices just described can continuously and directly measure acceleration in a form that is immediately useable (e.g., a chart recorder or an oscilliscope).
- They can, if specified, have very high frequency responses suitable for impact studies of helmets, face masks, matting, and other protective equipment.
- If proper mounting and fixation procedures are used, measurements will be very accurate.

Disadvantages.

- These types of measurement devices are feasible only for measuring single segments or bodies and so are inappropriate for assessing some human motions.
- They may cause an alteration of the subject's performance due to a need for fixation or because of size, weight, and need for cabling or telemetry.
- Attachment to soft tissues can cause discomfort and may lead to serious errors in measurement due to relative motion of the accelerometer and tissues.
- Absolute motion of the accelerometer is difficult to determine unless a six or nine accelerometer system is employed.
- The accelerometers combined with the necessary signal conditioning are relatively expensive.

ELECTROGONIOMETERS

Electrogoniometers (elgons) are devices that attach to the body and are capable of electrically measuring joint angles. Therefore, these devices may interfere or alter a subject's performance. Most models are designed for use in clinical settings, so this is not a problem. However, some have been used for sport research (e.g., Gollnick & Karpovitch, 1964; Klissouras & Karpovitch, 1967).

Electrogoniometers can be designed to measure rotations about one, two, or three axes and at almost any joint. Some commercially available models (CARS-UBC or MERU) (Figure 2.8) can measure triaxial rotations about the hip, knee, and ankle of both legs simultaneously—a total of 18 joint rotations (Cousins, 1975; Hannah, Cousins, & Foort, 1978).

Other design features include self-alignment (e.g., Cousins, 1975; Lamoreux, 1971) and intersection of the electrogoniometer's axes with the joint's axes (see Chao, 1978, Figure 2). Another model designed by Kinzel, Hillberry, Hall, Sickle, and Harvey (1972), is even capable of measuring the linear motion at a joint; however, this device requires a skeletal pin and is limited to cadaver, prosthetic, or animal research.

Advantages.

- Elgons can continuously and directly measure in one, two, or three dimensions, the joint rotations at one or more joints without expensive data collection or processing facilities.
- They are relatively inexpensive, easy to operate, reliable, and can provide data immediately.
- They can be used to measure bilateral rotations.

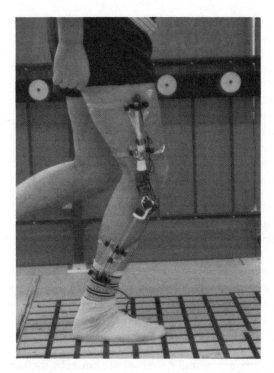

Figure 2.8 Electrogoniometer mounted for three-dimensional monitoring at knee joint.

Disadvantages.

- The wearing of these transducers may alter performance and problems may arise due to the need for connecting with recording devices or the need for telemetering outputs.
- They give information relative to the body and not to the absolute motion of joints, although some designs (Peat, Grahame, Fulford, & Quanbury, 1976) have partially overcome this problem.
- Finally, they present potential errors when the axes of the device do not coincide with those of the joint; however, some designs can overcome this problem or corrections can be made digitally (see Chao, 1978, 1980).

Interpretation of Test Results

The researcher must realize that all measured results will contain some component of error. This error component will limit the subsequent value that these measurements have in contributing to the kinetic model of the athletic performance. The error component of the raw kinematic data can result from such things as

- perspective error,
- digitization error,
- digitizer resolution,
- camera vibration,
- film analyzer distortion,
- instrument synchronization error,
- instrument calibration error, and
- error in identifying anatomical landmarks.

The amount of error in any measurement is dependent to a large extent on the test protocol as well as on the quality of the equipment used in the experiment. Thus any technique used for the collecting of kinematic data must be well validated beforehand.

The information content of kinematic data by itself is minimal. The information must be integrated into kinetic computations to really justify the time and effort used in its gathering process.

Kinematic Written Reports

The following experimental specifications must be included in any kinematic research report.

1. The actual kinematic parameters measured.
2. The proper SI units.
3. The measurement technique used in the research project. The description must be of sufficient depth to allow another lab to duplicate the experiment if necessary.
4. The smoothing and differentiation technique employed, if one is reporting the calculated derivatives of displacement data (i.e., velocity and acceleration).

The decision to use any measurement device for the collection of kinematic data must be made with knowledge of the purpose for which the results are to be used. If used in isolation, then the accuracy will be limited only to the device, the electronic amplification, and the recording equipment, and in some instances the ability of the researcher to mount and secure the equipment to reduce any artifact. If the data are further to be used as kinematic inputs to models or other derived information, then the processing of the raw data also becomes very important. To better understand how the data obtained from the techniques described in this chapter are used in further analysis, turn to the chapter on kinetics that follows.

3

Kinetics

MICHELINE GAGNON
GORDON ROBERTSON
ROBERT NORMAN

The subject matter in kinetics, the very complex and perhaps most extensive area of investigation in biomechanics, has been examined with respect to physical entities for hundreds if not thousands of years. Kinetics concerns the underlying reasons for movement rather than the results of movement, as kinematics does. The forces, energy, power, and efficiency involved in human movement provide for an understanding of motion on a more complex level. The use of modeling and other computer techniques is an integral part of any kinetic investigation. Consequently, a more in-depth discussion of the components of this subdiscipline is necessary.

In order to understand the study of kinetics with respect to human movement, a basic comprehension of the properties of the body and its parts is a prerequisite. Consequently, this chapter begins with a section on body segment parameters. The first section addresses this topic in some detail, considering the reasons for measuring, the things to be measured, the results obtained, and the shortcomings of the techniques and results. The second section of the chapter begins the detailed look at kinetics by examining forces, impulses, and momenta. Mechanical work and energy and efficiency will be discussed in the third section. As in chapter 2, techniques of testing will be discussed briefly.

Physical Properties of the Limbs and Total Body

The following properties of the limbs will be examined: mass or weight and the related parameters (volume and density), center of mass and center of volume, and moments of inertia. These properties will be defined and the units in the international system will be presented.

DEFINITIONS AND STANDARD UNITS

Mass, weight, and related parameters.   The *mass* (M) is a quantitative measure of inertia. It is the quantity of matter included in the body. The units are in kilograms (kg). The *density* (d) of a body is the mass per unit of volume: d = M/V. It is expressed in kilograms per meter cubed (kg/m^3).

The mass and weight can be measured for parts of the segment, for the entire segment, and for the total body. Procedures of summation may be used whenever appropriate.

Segmental and total body center of mass (or center of gravity).   The *center of gravity* (CG) is that point for which the moment about any axis of the resultant of the gravity force equals the sum of the moments about the same axis due to the elemental gravity forces (for a continuous distribution of matter) or due to the discrete gravity forces (for discrete point masses). In other words, the moments of a sum equals the sum of the moments of a body. This concept is called Varignon's theorem. If the coordinates of the center of gravity are designated by x, y, and z, and the total weight by W, the moment principle gives

$$\bar{x} = \frac{\int x dW}{W} \; ; \; \bar{y} = \frac{\int y dW}{W} \; ; \; \bar{z} = \frac{\int z dW}{W} \text{ (continuous)} \qquad (3\text{-}1)$$

or

$$\bar{x} = \frac{\Sigma x_i W_i}{\Sigma W_i} \; ; \; \bar{y} = \frac{\Sigma y_i W_i}{\Sigma W_i} \; ; \; \bar{z} = \frac{\Sigma z_i W_i}{\Sigma W_i} \text{ (discrete)} \qquad (3\text{-}2)$$

The point of application of the equivalent resultant gravitational force is called the center of gravity. More simply stated, the CG is an imaginary point at which all the mass of the body may be considered to be acting.

The center of mass (CM) coincides with the center of gravity and is obtained by interchanging W by M. The units for CM and CG are in meters (m).

Segmental mass moment of inertia.   The *mass moment of inertia* (I) is a measure of the inertial resistance of a body to rotation. It is expressed in two ways, depending on if the body is considered to be distributed continuously or if it is composed of discrete point masses.

The formula I = $\int r^2$ dm (for continuous distribution of matter) is used where dm represents an infinitesimal mass and r is the distance from such an element to the axis of rotation and orthogonal to this axis. This approach is generally adopted when the segment is assumed to represent known geometric shapes such as spheres and frustra of cone.

$$I = \sum m_i r_i^2 = d\sum V_i r_i^2 \text{ (for discrete point masses)} \qquad (3\text{-}3)$$

In this instance, the segment is generally assumed to be composed of several sections for which the masses and centers of masses can be approximated. The units are in kg • m^2.

The *parallel axis theorem* is a proof of the relation between the moment of inertia of a body about any axis and the moment of inertia with respect to a parallel axis through the center of mass (I_{CM}). This relation is expressed as $I = I_{CM} + Mh^2$ where h stands for the distance between the two axes and is orthogonal to these axes. This relation is useful when the researcher wants to evaluate the moment of inertia about a proximal of distal joint, if he or she knows the moment of inertia about its center of mass and the location of the center of mass.

The *radius of gyration* is the measure of mass distribution from the axis in question. It is expressed as $k = \sqrt{I/M}$. The units are in meters (m).

LIMITATIONS

The limitations inherent in the different techniques will be discussed under the section Testing Procedures. However, certain generalizations relative to the limitations involved in approximating the physical properties of the limb must be mentioned: (a) the validity problem remains for all techniques applied to living subjects, and (b) the validity of the measures obtained with cadavers remains questionable for their application to populations of living subjects.

PURPOSE FOR MEASURING

The analysis of human performance from cinematographic pictures shows the importance of determining the physical properties of the limbs. These properties constitute the basic information required for the simplest type of kinematic analysis such as depicting the patterns of displacement of the total body center of gravity. The properties also comprise the knowledge needed for a more complicated type of kinetic analysis implying modeling the body segments for the purpose of approximating the muscular torques at the joints and the transarticular reaction forces.

RELEVANCE

A few examples are illustrated in Table 3.1 to show the relationships between specific physical properties and movement parameters.

Table 3.1   Relationship Between Physical Properties and Movement Parameters

Movement Parameters	Physical Properties
Take-off and touch-down angle	Total body center of gravity and a specified point (toe, ankle)
Linear displacement of the body (on the ground or in flight)	Total body center of gravity relative to a reference point
Linear velocities	Kinematic formulae applied to CG displacement over time
Muscular torques and transarticular forces	Location of joint center (X, Y), location of the segmental CG (X, Y), segmental weight and mass moment of inertia about the joint center, and application of kinetic equations (via free body diagrams and mass-acceleration diagrams)
Body position in aquatic motions	Location of both the center of volume and center of gravity; the distance between these centers and the evaluation of the torque causing the lower part of the body to drop

TESTING PROCEDURES

In this section the various measurement techniques and methods will be examined. These procedures will be classified under the following items:

1. Mass (or weight) and related parameters
2. Center of mass (or center of gravity) and center of volume
3. Mass moments of inertia

Mass (or weight) and related parameters.   The determination of the total mass of the human body is an easy routine but that is not the case for the segmental masses. As a matter of fact, no direct means of recording this property in living subjects exists, and several types of approximations are suggested in the literature. Some approximations are derived from cadaver data, and some are based on specific techniques of approximation applied to living subjects.

Studies With Cadavers.   Dempster (1955) provided some norms on segmental weights derived from a sample of eight cadavers. The frozen segments were dissected and weighed; the weights were expressed as percentages relative to total body weight. This source of information is the one most currently used in biomechanics research.

Regression equations were also developed by Barter (1957) and Clauser, McConville, and Young (1969). Barter used different samples obtained by several authors for a total of 12 cadavers and expressed simple linear regression equations to predict the segmental weight as a function of total body weight. Clauser developed multiple linear regression equations to predict the segmental masses as a function of total body mass and developed specific anthropometric dimensions from a sample of 13 embalmed cadavers. The validity of these two types of regression equations was examined by Miller and Morrison (1975) with a sample of male athletes; Barter's regression equations tend to underestimate the total mass by an average of 2.03%, whereas Clauser's equations tend to overestimate it by 4.59%.

The problems related to these studies must be emphasized:

1. The sizes of the samples were small, and the regression equations' validity is questionable in these cases. Moreover, the samples were atypical with regard to the populations of athletes to which these norms and regression equations are applied (sex, age, morphology, etc.).
2. Different dissection techniques were used by the investigators.
3. Different procedures of conservation were adopted (fresh cadavers, frozen, or with added preservative). With preservatives, the changes that may be included in the biological tissues are not well substantiated (Clauser et al., 1969).
4. Losses in tissue and body fluids are encountered during dissection.
5. Losses in body tissue (degeneration) are associated with the state of health preceding death.

Studies with living subjects.   The three types of approach generally encountered in the literature are the reaction change method, the relation $M = Vd$, and regression equations. The *reaction change method* was used by Drillis and Contini (1966). It consists of approximating the segmental weight by measuring the change of force reaction when a segment is moved from an original to a final position. In this technique, the subject lies on a board that is positioned on two fulcra. Force measurements are recorded at one of the fulcra either by a scale or force transducers.

The problems associated with this technique are that the center of mass must be approximated, and muscular contraction presumably does not induce differences in mass distribution in the moving segment and in the adjacent stationary segments. This hypothesis may be questionable: Clauser et al. (1969) mentioned that the belly of the muscle can be displaced by as much as 2 to 3 cm during muscular contraction.

The *relation* $M = Vd$ is used when the segmental mass is approximated by the product of volume and segmental density. The precision of this measurement depends on two types of determination that will be discussed:

Approximation of segmental density.   Generally, the segmental density is assumed to remain constant throughout the segment. According to Rodrigue (1981), this hypothesis is not tenable; she found that the segmental density of the forearm in cadavers increased in the extremities and decreased in the central part of the segment. Presently, the information with regard to segmental density is obtained from cadavers (Dempster, 1955).

A few studies are available regarding the densities of biological tissues. It is apparent that the densities of skin, fat, and muscle show only slight variations within the subject and between subjects (Clauser et al., 1969; Fidanza & Anderson, 1953; Leider & Buncke, 1954). On the other hand, the density of bone varies considerably according to age and sex, the type of bone (spongy or compact), the section of bone (transverse or longitudinal), and the type of preparation (dried fully or partially saturated with water). The reader is referred to the studies by Atkinson and Wheatherell (1967), Lindahl and Lindgren (1967), and Wall, Chatterji, and Jeffery (1972, 1979).

Approximation of segmental volume.   The easiest and most precise method to evaluate the segmental volume is by *immersion* (Gagnon & Rodrigue, 1979; Katch, Weltman, & Gold, 1974; Little & Jessup, 1977). However, this method appears extremely difficult to apply to proximal segments such as the arm and thigh and to the head, neck, and trunk.

The volume can also be approximated by *geometrical models* in which each segment is represented by geometrical forms such as spheres, cylinders, and frustra of cone (Hanavan, 1964; Kalwicki, Schlei, & Vergamini, 1962; Whitsett, 1963). These models were not validated with respect to segmental properties. Hanavan's model has been currently used in biomechanics research. Gagnon and Rodrigue (1979) validated the forearm model developed by Hanavan and found that this model tends to underestimate the segmental volume by an average of 15%. A problem of conformity was apparent, especially in the region neighboring the elbow. They further refined this model by dividing the segment with five frustra of cone. The conformity problem was still present but to a lesser extent; the segmental volume was underestimated by an average of 5% when compared to results from immersion.

Other types of models have been developed in which the segmental cross sections are assumed to be represented by ellipses whose diameters are measured from two orthogonal photographs (Gagnon & Rodrigue, 1979; Jensen, 1978; Weinbach, 1938). Gagnon and Rodrigue found no significant differences between the volumes measured by this technique and by immersion.

Hatze (1980) also presented a technique for determining segmental volumes using a finite element approach. He took into consideration the relative distribution of biological tissues determined by Dempster (1955) for one cadaver that was dissected into slices of 1 in. Moreover, Hatze provided the tissue densities obtained by Clauser on several samples taken in four cadavers as input data. This method requires a somewhat lengthy procedure (approximately 1-1/2 hr), as the measurements are taken directly on the subjects; however, the results obtained are highly consistent with other computational techniques.

Some *regression equations* were developed by Zatsiorsky and Seluyanov (1983, 1985) in the U.S.S.R. from a sample of 100 living men ranging from 19 to 35 years of age. The physical properties including mass, center of gravity, mass moment of inertia, and radius of gyration were obtained from the gamma-scanner method, which was previously validated on cadavers and biological objects. Zatsiorsky and Seluyanov used a finite element approach, and the surface density (cross sections) could be evaluated by measuring the intensity of the gamma radiation beam before and after its passage through the layer of material. They mentioned that the radiation dose was well under the permissible dose. It is questionable if this technique could be applied in North American society. However, the study is a very useful and valuable source of information.

Center of mass (or gravity) and center of volume.   Distinguishing between the total body and segmental properties is important. When the segmental center of mass is discussed, reference will be made to studies with cadavers and with living subjects.

Total body's center of gravity and center of volume.   A technique was developed by Gagnon and Montpetit (1981) to measure the location of the body's center of volume for different body positions and states of expiration. The method involves the application of hydrostatic procedures and allows the determination of other properties such as the location of the center of gravity, the body volume, and density. These properties become valuable to detect some elements that may be pertinent in swimming performance. This technique is limited in the sense that it can be applied only when the body is in a static state.

Segmental center of mass in cadavers.   Very precise information can be obtained from techniques applied to cadavers. The segments are dissected and the center of gravity is usually determined by means of the reaction board technique. Dempster (1955) developed norms by which the location of the segmental center of gravity is expressed as a percentage relative to the segment length. Clauser et al. (1969) developed multiple linear regression equations to predict the location of the segmental center of gravity as a function of several anthropometric dimensions. The problems associated with cadaver data were already mentioned in the section relative to mass determination. The main difficulty concerns the validity of Dempster's norms and Clauser's regression equations when applied to different populations of living subjects.

Segmental center of mass in living subjects.   The three types of experimental approaches encountered in the literature are *immersion, geometrical approximations* or *models,* and *regression equations.* The *immersion* technique has been used by Cleveland (1955) to approximate the segmental center of mass. The volume of the segment is first determined, and then the point corresponding to its midvolume is identified. The main hypothesis is that the center of mass coincides with the center of volume.

This hypothesis of coincidence between the center of mass and the center of volume needs to be tested. Little research is available. Bernstein (1930) reported that for all practical purposes these two centers do coincide; however, no data are available for examination. Clauser et al. (1969) found these centers to differ by an average of 5% of the segmental length in cadavers. The errors were in a constant direction: The center of mass was always closer to the proximal joint than the center of volume was. Rodrigue (1981) found that the two centers differ by an average of only 1% in cadaver forearms. More research is needed to investigate these disparate views.

The center of mass (or center of volume) is also approximated by *geometrical models* of the entire segment (Hanavan, 1964) or parts of the segment (Gagnon & Rodrigue, 1979; Hatze, 1980; Jensen, 1978). When the entire segment is considered, Varignon's theorem is applied for a continuous distribution of matter. When the segment is analyzed by parts, Varignon's theorem refers to discrete point masses. The same hypothesis is made regarding the coincidence of the center of volume and the center of mass.

Regression equations were also developed by Zatsiorsky and Seluyanov (1983) for the prediction of the segmental center of mass. This study and its limitations were presented in the section Mass (or Weight) and Related Parameters.

Mass moments of inertia.   The segmental mass moments of inertia were investigated in cadavers and in living subjects. The techniques of investigation and their limitations are presented.

Studies with cadavers.   Dempster (1955) used the *compound pendulum* to measure the moments of inertia about the joints in dissected cadavers. The formula used is expressed as

$$I = \frac{MghT^2}{4\pi^2} \qquad (3\text{-}4)$$

where T stands for the period of oscillation, M is the segmental mass, g is the acceleration due to gravity, and h is the distance from the segmental center of mass to the joint or axis of rotation. The evaluation of the moment of inertia depends on three independent types of measures that can decrease the level of precision associated with this property. Dempster reported the specific values recorded on his sample of cadavers. However, these values were not in a form appropriate for application in living subjects. Plagenhoef (1971) worked through Dempster's data on moments of inertia and mass and expressed the radius of gyration of each segment as a percentage of the segmental length relative to the proximal and distal joints. These norms are the only ones known with respect to radii of gyration. From these values and mass data, it is possible to approximate the moments of inertia in living subjects.

Some regression equations have also been developed to relate the total body moment of inertia to body weight (Clauser et al., 1969). The regression analysis of moments of inertia versus weight yielded correlation coefficients ranging from 0.77 to 0.98.

Studies with living subjects.   Several types of techniques were used with living subjects including geometrical models, regression equations, the *compound pendulum method*, the *quick-release method*, and the *suspension method*.

Geometrical models were used to represent the segment as a whole or by parts. Hanavan (1964) and Woolley (1967) applied their models to the whole segment. In these models, the computational approach for a continuous distribution of matter is used to evaluate the mass moments of inertia. Hanavan undertook validation procedures by comparing the total body moment of inertia about specified axes obtained experimentally from compound pendulum methods and obtained mathematically from the modeled segments. The error distribution among the different segments was not determined. The error on total body moment of inertia was within 10%.

Geometrical models were also applied to parts of the segment (Gagnon & Rodrigue, 1979; Hatze, 1980; Jensen, 1978). In these cases, the computational methods of moment of inertia for discrete point masses are used. Hatze (1980) presented the most refined model in which each of 17 segments was decomposed into finite elements of known geometrical structure (not necessarily symmetrical). Each element was then assigned its own density value. This model took into consideration the relative distribution of biological tissues (from Dempster, 1955) and their respective densities (from Clauser, 1969). The moment of inertia mathematically computed by the modeled segment is consistent with the moment of inertia obtained experimentally from suspension techniques. The majority of these approaches still rely on the very uncertain assumptions that the segmental masses and centers of mass may be accurately determined and that the segmental density is uniform along the segment and is known.

Regression equations were developed by Zatsiorsky and Seluyanov (1983) to predict the principal moments of inertia about the three orthogonal axes at the joint as a function of anthropometric measurements. They also gave the radii of gyration, which were expressed as percentages relative to segmental lengths.

The *compound pendulum* method is mentioned only for purposes of information because it is not used presently. Hill (1940) used this method with one subject to evaluate the forearm and hand moment of inertia about the elbow. This method implies several types of measurement as mentioned previously with studies on cadavers. However, one important problem is also associated with this technique: Complete relaxation of the subject may be difficult to obtain, and muscular torques may be induced during oscillations. Passive viscoelastic torques may also be present.

The *quick-release method* was used by Bouisset and Pertuzon (1967) and by Cavanagh and Gregor (1974). This method is based on the following relationships:

$$\tau = I\alpha \qquad (3\text{-}5)$$

where τ is the torque exerted by the subject when in a static position, and α is the angular acceleration recorded at the moment of release. Cavanagh and Gregor (1974) found that a large disparity was present in the values of moment of inertia when the position of force application was varied along the segment (Figure 3.1). This technique must be refined to produce reliable data.

A newer method called the *suspension method* was developed by Hatze (1975). It was based on the theory of damped oscillation of a system about its equilibrium position. Simultaneous measurements of the moment of inertia, the damping coefficient, and location of the center of mass of a body segment could be obtained. Later, Hayes and Hatze (1977) developed procedures to estimate the passive elastic torque function and the passive viscous torque function of the muscles and connective tissues spanning the joint. They also assessed whether myotatic reflex activity could bias the value of the torque contributed by passive viscous elements. These studies were the only ones encountered in the literature in which the elastic and viscous properties were assessed and eliminated from the moment of inertia determination. However, this method presented certain limitations in that the segmental mass and the segmental center of rotation must be approximated. The value of the moment of inertia as determined by this method is consistent with computational methods.

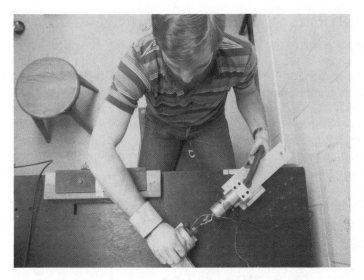

Figure 3.1 Quick release system using force transducer, accelerometer, and electromagnet to measure the moment of inertia of the forearm.

INTERPRETATION OF TEST RESULTS

The information provided about the segmental properties must be interpreted with care: Full validity of these measures has not been demonstrated. Slight errors associated with a single property of a given segment may not be too critical, but when the kinetic analyses imply the approximation of several of these properties for all body segments, the total error may be substantial. More research is needed to evaluate the relative effects of these errors on the kinematic and kinetic parameters associated with human motion.

Forces, Impulse, and Momentum

Dynamics is that branch of mechanics that concerns the motion of bodies under the action of forces. Dynamics includes two aspects: kinematics, the study of motion without reference to the forces that cause motion, and *kinetics*, which relates the action of forces on bodies to their resulting motions. In this chapter, the kinetic parameters will be examined: *force and torque, impulse and momentum, pressure, mechanical energy, work, efficiency*, and *power*.

DEFINITIONS AND STANDARD UNITS

The *force* (F) is the vector quantity necessary to cause a change in momentum. When an unbalanced force acts on a body, the body accelerates in the direction of that force. The acceleration is directly proportional to the unbalanced force and inversely proportional to the mass of the body (a = F/M). The units of force are in Newtons (N) where $1\,N = 1\,kg \cdot m/s^2$.

Torque or *moment of force* (τ) consists of the product of force and the perpendicular distance from the axis of rotation to the line of action of the force (lever arm). It is expressed in Newton-meters (N • m).

Linear impulse is the product of force and time; the *linear momentum* is the product of mass and the change in linear velocity. The total linear impulse on a mass in a given direction equals the corresponding change in linear momentum in the same direction.

$$\int F_x dt = M (V_{f_x} - V_{i_x}) \tag{3-6}$$

$$\int F_y dt = M (V_{f_x} - V_{i_y}) \tag{3-7}$$

$$\int F_z dt = M (V_{f_x} - V_{i_z}) \tag{3-8}$$

The units of measurements for linear impulse are Newton-second (N • s) and those for linear momentum are kilogram-meter per second (kg • m/s).

Impact refers to a special case of impulse. It consists of the collision between two or more bodies and is characterized by the generation of relatively large contact forces that act over a very short interval of time.

Angular impulse is the product of moment of force about the point of rotation and time. The point of rotation may be located at the mass center (free flight) or at some other location. The *angular momentum* is the product of moment of inertia (I) and angular velocity (ω). The total change in angular momentum attributed to angular impulse corresponds to the change of Iω during the time course of impulse.

$$\int \Sigma M_{cm} dt = [(I\omega)_f - (I\omega)_i]_{cm} \text{ about the mass center} \tag{3-9}$$

$$\int \Sigma M_o dt = [(I\omega)_f - (I\omega)_i]_o \text{ about any axis passing through O} \tag{3-10}$$

The units of angular impulse are expressed in Newton-meter-seconds (N • m • s) and those of angular momentum are in kilogram-meter^2 per second (kg • m^2/s).

Pressure is defined as the amount of force acting per unit area. The force is the one acting perpendicularly to the area. The units are the pascal (Pa), which equals 1 N/m².

LIMITATIONS

The researcher is usually interested in measuring ground reaction forces, joint reaction forces, muscular forces and moments of forces, impact forces on sport equipment (shoes, tennis rackets, etc.), and pressure distribution. Some limitations are inherent in the determination of these parameters for the human body. These limitations will be presented in more detail later. However, the general problems associated with these measurements are briefly exposed here.

- The net muscular torques can be approximated reasonably well through cinematographic procedures. The accuracy of the measurements and their validity depend on such factors as the validity of the basic information concerning the physical properties of the limbs and the validity of numerical differentiation procedures adopted to approximate velocities and accelerations from displacement time data. Moreover, the error increases with the number of links included in the analyses.
- The approximation of muscular forces still remains a major problem in biomechanics. These forces cannot be directly quantified by means of electromyography techniques except in relatively simple (single joint) or very slow movements over restricted ranges of joint angles. However, progress is being made in research in this area. The approximation of muscular forces by means of modeling combined with cinematographic procedures presents the same limitations as those mentioned for muscular torques. Additionally, these forces have the limitations regarding supplementary assumptions such as the direction of force, its point of application relative to the joint center, and the absence of co-contraction. The same problem applies in the evaluation of effective bone-on-bone contact forces at the joint because the evaluation requires valid information concerning the muscular forces.
- Ground reaction forces and impact forces on some pieces of equipment can be determined with relatively high accuracy. The limitations are those associated with the dynamic performance characteristics of the force transducers.
- Pressure distribution measurements present some limitations related to the technological development, which is still unsatisfactory.

Measurements of *linear and angular impulses* are limited only by the precision inherent in the force transducers (generally a force platform) and by the validity of numerical integration procedures of force as a function of time.

The determination of *linear momentum* can be made very accurately when the initial velocity of the subject is null. Otherwise, the critical factor is the one associated with the evaluation of that initial velocity; in that case, numerical differentiation procedures are generally adopted, and a high level of uncertainty may be associated with this value. The problem is much more complex when the angular momentum is evaluated. It depends (a) on the approximation of the total body's moment of inertia associated with large uncertainties (see Physical Properties of the Limbs and Total Body) and (b) on complex mathematical procedures to evaluate the angular velocity of the body.

PURPOSE FOR MEASURING

The kinetic analysis is important in the evaluation of sport performance. The analysis allows the researcher to evaluate the causes of deficient or superior performance of motion, to present a diagnosis, and to formulate pertinent recommendations with regard to training. These measurements, especially impact forces and pressure distribution, are also highly significant in evaluating risk factors associated with specific sport motions, different types of sport equipment (such as shoes and helmets), and different sport environments (such as the quality of floor surfaces and walls).

RELEVANCE

A few sport applications will be presented to illustrate the relevance in measuring the kinetic parameters.

Muscular forces and moments of force.   The patterns of muscular forces or moments of force as a function of time provide informative data regarding the level of exertion by the athlete during performance. The patterns also provide data regarding the relative efficiency of motion reflected either by the presence of parasite contractions in certain muscular groups (excessive co-contraction of both the agonist and antagonist muscles) or by phases in which contraction in the agonist and antagonist muscles (e.g., the recovery leg during running) is absent.

Joint reaction forces.   The measurement of joint reaction forces can be useful in evaluating the importance of forces tolerated by the body during the performance of activities involving large impacts such as those encountered in the triple jump, the hurdle, and the touchdown following the smash in volleyball. These joint reaction forces may be minimized with suitable techniques and sport equipment.

Ground reaction forces.   Ground reaction forces are usually measured by means of force plates. They are required to further evaluate joint reaction forces. They are generally combined with cinematographic information about the subject's center of mass. Therefore, the magnitudes of force, their directions, and their locations relative to the center of mass are used to evaluate the deficiencies in motion.

Impulses.   The impulse, especially the linear impulse, is often evaluated from ground reaction force measurements. The calculation of impulse at successive, small time intervals may be combined with mass data to picture the velocity development during performance. For instance, the relative contribution of the rear and front foot to propulsion during the track start may be obtained by comparing the total impulse exerted on each starting block.

Momenta.   From measurements of linear momentum, the researcher is interested in the evaluation of linear velocity development during the performance (e.g., comparison of different track start techniques and comparison between sprinters of different ability) or by the final velocity that results from impulse (e.g., the takeoff in long jump) and regulates the trajectory during the phase of nonsupport. The angular momentum of the total body is usually measured to examine the effects of segmental motions on body rotation and position (e.g., diving and the long jump). This approach is generally used in computer simulations of the airborne phase of motion.

Pressure distribution.   This measurement allows the researcher to examine the areas of greater force concentration during support. This type of information becomes very useful in improving the design of sport equipment. For instance, the evaluation of pressure distribution under the foot in running provides substantial information to evaluate the running technique, to improve the experimental design of shoe evaluation, and to provide criteria for improving the shoe design.

MEASUREMENT TECHNIQUES AND TESTS

This section contains an overview of the various measurement techniques and tests, with comments on their specific strengths and weaknesses, for the evaluation of kinetic parameters.

Muscular forces and moments, joint reaction forces.   The evaluation of the internal parameters associated with human motion such as *muscular* *forces and moments of force,* and *joint reaction forces* constitutes a complex task requiring several basic pieces of information including description of the kinematics of motion (displacement, velocity, and acceleration for translation and rotation). This information is obtained by means of cinematographical techniques and numerical smoothing and differentiation procedures. Although substantial progress has been made in the area of numerical analysis applied to human motion, more research is needed to validate these procedures for complex sport motions.

The values of the physical properties of the limbs (masses, centers of mass, moments of inertia, and joint centers) are also basic pieces of information, and can be obtained using the methods or using the results directly that are available in the literature (see section on physical properties of the limbs). These values are associated with uncertainties, and full validity has not yet been demonstrated. A knowledge of muscular attachment sites relative to the joint centers and direction of muscular pull is also important. These data are required for determining muscular forces and joint reaction forces, but they are not required if only the muscular moments are evaluated. This type of information is provided from anatomical studies.

The evaluation of ground reaction forces and their location relative to the joint centers is also necessary information for evaluating human motion. This information is obtained by means of a force platform and is valid provided the force platform performance characteristics are demonstrated. These forces are required when the support limb is analyzed. However, the forces are not required for analysis of segments for which support is not provided. Generally, any external force applied by the human on his or her environment must be determined.

The muscular forces and moments and joint reaction forces are determined by means of free body diagrams using the method of statics or dynamics according to the type of application. This model is called a linked-segment model (Winter, 1979a). In Figure 3.2 procedures are shown

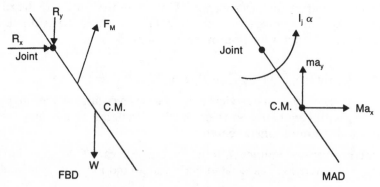

Figure 3.2 Free-body diagram of terminal segment.

for a planar motion of a segment free of the ground (e.g., the foot during the swing phase).

Dynamic equations for planar motion are:

$$\Sigma F_x = Ma_x \tag{3-11}$$

$$\Sigma F_y = Ma_y \tag{3-12}$$

$$\Sigma T_j = I_j\alpha \tag{3-13}$$

Unless the direction of the muscular force and its location relative to the joint center are determined, the problem will be indeterminate. Moreover, the problem has already been simplified by assuming that only one muscle was acting in that motion, and clearly, the problem will become much more complex when several muscles or muscle groups are simultaneously active. To remove the indetermination, the muscular force is resolved into an equivalent force at the joint and a couple.

This model has been used by Boccardi, Pedotti, Rodano, and Santambrogio, 1981; Cappozzo, Leo, and Pedotti, 1975; Cavanagh and Gregor, 1975; Robertson and Winter, 1980; and Winter, 1980. The strengths and weaknesses associated with this approach are important. With this model, the researcher can evaluate the resultant muscular moment about the joint. The investigator can also identify if that resultant moment is predominantly eccentric or concentric according to the direction of the angular velocity of the limb relative to the direction of the moment of force (Robertson & Winter, 1980). However, it is necessary to mention the most important limitations associated with the model.

Optimization techniques are used that involve the assumption of optimal coordination, which in turn implies that only one muscular group, either the agonist or the antagonist group, is active at any moment during the motion. As a matter of fact, an unlimited number of combinations of agonist and antagonist muscular moments could produce a given value of resultant muscular moment, but their relative contributions cannot be dissociated. For instance, the resultant muscular moment could be null and the motion interpreted as being ballistic, but in reality the motion could be attributed to equal agonist and antagonist moments. However, optimization techniques are believed to be justified in the analysis of certain highly controlled motions such as gait or motions executed by elite performers. These techniques remain questionable when applied to the analysis of motions that are not mastered or that are associated with pathological defects. Another limitation is that the joint reaction forces so determined are not meaningful because the components attributed to muscular contractions must be added to their external counterparts to provide valid measures of bone-on-bone contact forces (Winter, 1979a). The contribution to joint reaction moments by such structures as ligaments is considered negligible, another limitation. This hypothesis needs to be validated for application to strenuous types of sport activities.

Some other models have been developed to calculate the loads on a given joint and the contraction levels of muscles. Most of the models were developed for applications in the field of ergonomics to quasi-static activities (Andersson, Ortengren, & Schultz, 1980; Chaffin, 1969; McNeill, Warwick, Andersson, & Schultz, 1980; Schultz & Andersson, 1981). Schultz and Andersson (1981) discussed the assumptions involved in these models. First, quasi-static motion may be assumed in the case where the inertial forces (Ma) and inertial moments (Iα) produced are of little significance when compared with forces and moments needed for equilibrium. As a matter of fact, few quantitative studies of dynamic effects in athletic and nonathletic activities are available.

A second assumption is that when all muscular forces and their locations relative to the joint center are examined, the problem becomes statically indeterminate. This problem can be solved through the use of optimization techniques; the simplest of these techniques is probably linear programming (Dantzig, 1968). In that case, the quantity to be optimized must be chosen. For instance, in a study on the lumbar spine, the researcher may choose to minimize the compression on the lumbar vertebrae and to impose some constraints, specifically that the muscle tensions may not be negative and may not exceed a reasonable level. The solution routine automatically selects them, and in this solution, the muscles contract with their maximum allowed intensity. Schultz and Andersson reasoned that the objective function choice does not seem very important in maximum exertion activities because every muscle will contribute at maximum or near maximum intensity no matter what the objective function is. But in submaximal physical efforts, different objective functions can yield different estimates of muscle tensions. More research is needed to determine what choices the neuromuscular system makes when it has several options available for task performance. Assumptions must be made with regard to muscle site attachments and the direction of pull. The contribution to joint reaction moments by the ligaments is also considered negligible. This hypothesis may be tenable for activities of low intensity but remains questionable when high levels of exertion are involved.

The validation procedures of internal force estimates include measurements of myoelectric activity. This validation is only partial. The correlation between EMG activity and the predicted value of muscular force may be found, but the EMG activity does not provide quantitative information concerning the numerical value of force unless combined with calibration procedures such as those with isometric force and with the effects of muscle length and velocity. Compression forces at the joint may be validated by means of internal pressure measurements (e.g., the intradiscal pressure). This validation is also partial and based on correlation measures. The pressure measure at one given point may not be used to represent the total pressure applied on the joint and the subsequent total compression load.

In spite of these difficulties and because the range of loads experienced is so large, even a rough estimate of the loads generated by an activity will be sufficient for solutions of practical problems. The compression load on the lumbar spine, for instance, may be near zero in a lying position, 400 N while standing, and 4000 N in a strenuous type of activity (Schultz & Andersson, 1981).

Ground reaction forces and pressure distribution. *Ground reaction forces* are measured by means of force platforms (Figure 3.3). The technology of force platform design has evolved considerably in the last decade. Several investigators have chosen to have the platform designed for their own applications (Gagnon, 1978b; Payne, Slater, & Telford, 1968; Pelisse, 1979; Wilkerson & Cooper, 1979; and others). On the other hand, many types of manufactured platforms exist. One that is currently used in biomechanics research is the Kistler multicomponent measuring platform, type 9281 A 11; the transducers consist of quartz elements (piezoelectric effect) mounted under high pre-stress. It allows the measurement of three orthogonal components of any force acting on the platform, the coordinates of the instantaneous point of force application, and the torque with respect to an axis normal to the platform. The performance characteristics are described in the Newsletter (Vol. 5) of the Force Platform Group, I.S.B. (1978). The characteristics are high sensitivity and linearity, low

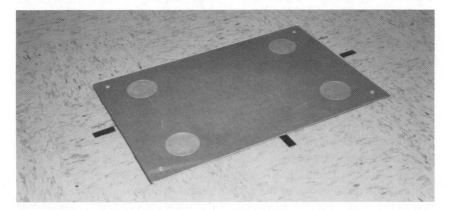

Figure 3.3 ''Kistler'' force platform.

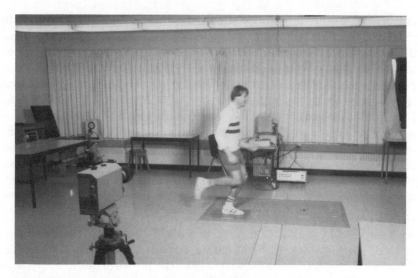

Figure 3.4 "AMTI" force plate used with 16mm camera.

hysteresis and cross-talk, and a very high natural frequency of 1 kHz. Measurement of quasi-static motions such as posture is apparently possible with this type of platform, but whether the discharge time constant is sufficiently large to provide valid data for this type of application is questionable. It is known that the signal discharges when piezoelectric transduction elements are used. Therefore, for this type of application, it seems more appropriate to use strain-gauged force platforms. Other manufactured platforms such as the AMTI 6-component biomechanical platform described in the Newsletter (Vol. 10) of the Force Platform Group, I.S.B. (1980) and the Amtech-Cook model OR6-2 multicomponent platform described in the Newsletter (Vol. 5) of the Force Platform Group, I.S.B. (1978) are also used. These two force platforms include strain gauges as transducers and allow the measurements of the three components of a force and the three torques about the three orthogonal axes of the platform (Figure 3.4). Both types of platform present high performance characteristics. The piezoelectric platforms present an advantage over the strain-gauged platforms in that they are less sensitive to temperature effects and can be operated at a very wide range of temperature. However, for most types of applications involving indoor activities both types of platforms may be used.

In designing or buying a force platform, the researcher should have in mind the dimensions of the platform and the problems related to targeting the surface of the platform. Valid measures of forces are related to adequate sensitivity, low threshold, high linearity, low hysteresis, low cross-talk between the different axes, elimination of interference associated with cable aberrations, electrical inductance, and temperature and humidity variations. The amplifier must be stable and linear and provide adequate gain. To choose an appropriate recording system matching the transducer in frequency response, the platform must provide high stiffness and high natural frequency and be located so that the vibrations are removed. These characteristics are described in chapter 5 under Recommended Procedures for Force Platforms and Pressure Platforms.

The major limitation of the conventional force platforms is that they provide information only about the center of pressure distribution (location of the point of application of the resultant force), and the pattern of pressure distribution cannot be determined by these means. Recently, several investigators applied their efforts in designing pressure platforms to measure the distribution of pressure at discrete locations beneath the foot. Scranton and McMaster (1976) measured the momentary distribution of forces under the foot by employing a liquid crystal display; however, the photographic display was not used for quantitative analyses. Arcan and Brull (1976) introduced an optical device for pressure measurement in which the interference rings were generated at discrete locations beneath a transparent surface. The normal force was determined by measuring the fringe diameter using a suitable calibration curve, but the problem associated with this technique is that the diameter of the ring is a nonlinear function of the local pressure. Hennig and Nichol (1978) constructed a pressure platform with a matrix of condenser elements linked to a similar matrix of light-emitting diodes. The light density depends on the force dependent impedance of the capacitors, and the main problem is associated with the recording of low density light signals. Cavanagh and Michiyoshi (1980) used a device similar to the one described by Arcan and Bull (1976). Their results on both static and dynamic calibrations showed the limitations of this technique for providing valid measures of pressure distribution: The static calibration indicated that a considerable change occurred in the gradient of the curve diameter of the ring versus pressure at higher levels, and the dynamic calibration indicated that an attenuation of approximately 15% of the peak values of pressure was present and a phase lag occurred during the decay of force input. They brought a substantial development in the method for displaying the data both visually (animated movie) and numerically. Hennig, Cavanagh, and MacMillan (1980) developed a pressure platform with piezoceramics used as transducer elements. Their initial experiments showed that this technique provides high linearity and low hysteresis, high response frequency, and high resolution.

The pressure platforms are designed to provide information about the distribution of pressure along discrete points beneath the foot. This consists of the distribution of forces over the area of contact. The force considered is the one normal to the area. Therefore, the shear forces tangential to the area are ignored in all the preceding designs. If shear forces are required along with the pressure distribution, the researcher should make a design combining a force platform over which a pressure plate would be positioned. This was attempted by Draganich, Andriacchi, Strongwater, and Galante (1980).

Impulses and momenta. *Linear* and *angular impulses* generated by the subject during propulsion on the ground may be easily determined from force platform measurements and integration procedures.

$$\int F_x dt; \quad \int F_y dt; \quad \int F_z dt; \text{ (linear impulse)} \tag{3-14}$$

$$\int M_{CG_x} dt; \quad \int M_{CG_y} dt; \quad \int M_{CG_z} dt; \text{ (angular impulse)} \tag{3-15}$$

These determinations are valid (a) if the force platform measurements are valid when the performance characteristics are adequate for the application under consideration, (b) if proper integration procedures are used (short sampling time and precise time measurements required), and (c) if the center of gravity can be determined with sufficient precision for the evaluation of angular impulse about the center of gravity. These limitations are discussed in the section, Physical Properties of the Limbs and Total Body.

The change in *linear momentum* ($\int F dt = M [v_f - v_i]$) can be determined from the information relative to linear impulse. Because the mass of the subject is constant, and provided the initial velocity v_i is known, the researcher can measure the final velocity v_f reached by the subject at any moment during the motion and resulting from the impulse. In this manner it is possible to trace the curve of velocity as a function of time during the impulse. The final velocity at the end of total impulse becomes a specific and interesting element of information because it may be used to predict the linear characteristics of flight (when applicable). The limitation of the technique is associated with the measurement of initial velocity before the subject strikes the platform. The initial velocity is assumed to be null when the subject is initially at rest such as in the sprint start (Gagnon, 1978a). Otherwise, the initial velocity must be evaluated by some other means, usually by cinematographical techniques from the path of the center of gravity prior to touchdown on the platform. No studies are reported in the literature in which this aspect was of concern.

Similarly, angular impulse is used to provide the measurement of the change in *angular momentum*.

$$\int \tau_{CG} dt = I_f\omega_f - I_i\omega_i \qquad (3\text{-}16)$$

The evaluation of angular impulse is complicated by the fact that the moment of inertia of the body about its center of mass may vary with the segmental positions in time and also that the initial angular velocity must be determined. When the initial angular velocity is null, the total momentum developed at takeoff is determined by integration of the moments of force applied on the force platform as a function of time. This integration requires the knoweldge of the magnitudes of force and their lever arms relative to the center of mass. This method was presented by Ramey (1974) for application to the long jump takeoff. Ramey apparently assumed that the initial angular momentum was null, a hypothesis that may be questionable in that type of motion.

Angular momentum may also be calculated directly from input data obtained by cinematography techniques. This approach was essentially used for applications to the airborne phase in diving (Miller, 1970; Grieve, Miller, Mitchelson, Paul, & Smith, 1975), in long jump (Ramey, 1973, 1974; Ramey & Yang, 1981), and in high jump (Dapena, 1981). In these cases, the assumption is made relative to the conservation of angular momentum (friction is assumed negligible). Miller used a four-segment model and therefore her approach can be used only for limited motions in two dimensions. She used the following relationships:

$$
\begin{aligned}
H^{s/cs} &= \text{a constant} \\
&= H^{B_1/c_1} + H^{B_2/c_2} + \ldots + H^{B_n/c_n} \\
&\quad + H^{c_1/cs} + H^{c_2/cs} + \ldots + H^{c_n/cs}
\end{aligned}
\qquad (3\text{-}17)
$$

Where H is angular momentum: $B_1, B_2 \ldots B_n$ represents the n interconnected rigid bodies or segments, $c_1 \ldots c_n$ are the mass centers of the n segments, s indicates the system as a whole, and cs is the mass center of the system. The approach is based on the dynamics of space motion for rigid bodies. The segmental angular positions were defined by Euler's angles. This model was later used by Ramey (1973) and extended to nine body segments. Hay, Wilson, and Dapena (1976) discussed the sources of error inherent in this approach: (a) a systematic error in the angular momentum may arise if the moment of inertia values are inappropriate, especially for the trunk segment; (b) the authors reported that when segment masses calculated from Barter's (1957) regression formula and proportions calculated from Clauser et al.'s (1969) mean data were substituted for Dempster's data (1955) used in this study, the angular momentum increased by approximately 30%.

Very few models have been proposed for the study of angular momentum in more general motions performed in tridimensional space. Ramey and Yang (1981) used a nine-body segments model where the trunk served as the reference to which the motion of all the other body segments was specified. However, this model could easily be extended to a more comprehensive body segment human model. The motions under study were those occurring during a free-fall, but the procedures included the effects of external forces at the initial stage. The equation of motion was developed using the principle of conservation of angular momentum referred to the mass center of the nine-body segment system. In this approach three Cartesian systems must be defined: (a) an inertial reference system, (b) a Cartesian system attached to the main body (trunk and head) located at its center of mass and whose axes are aligned with the principal axes of that body, and (c) a Cartesian system located at the center of mass of the body segment and with its axes aligned with the principal axes of the body segment (eight such systems are required for the eight body segments). The angular momentum of the nine-segment system with reference to its center of mass is written as

$$\overline{H} = \overline{\overline{I_o}} \cdot \omega_o + \sum_{k=1}^{8} \overline{\overline{I_k}} \cdot (\overline{\omega_o} + \overline{\omega_k}) + M_o \overline{R} \times \dot{\overline{R}} + \sum_{k=1}^{8} M_k [(\overline{\varrho_k} - \overline{R}) \times (\dot{\overline{\varrho}} - \dot{\overline{R}})] \tag{3-18}$$

where I_o is the moment of inertia of the main body (trunk plus head with respect to the principal axes of the system attached to its center of mass; I_k is the moment of inertia of the body segment relative to the principal axes of the system attached to the main body; ω_o is the absolute angular velocity of the main body; ω_k is the angular velocity of the body segment relative to the main body; ϱ_k is the position vector of the segmental center of mass relative to the center of mass of the main body; R the position vector of the system mass center relative to the center of mass of the main body; and the dot above the bar ($\dot{-}$) denotes vector derivatives with respect to the inertial reference system. Three-axis Euler angles must be used to describe the orientations. This model was used to evaluate the effects of prescribed relative body motions on the orientation of the human body during free-fall. However, this model was not validated.

A similar approach was used by Dapena (1981), who examined the discrepancies between the simulated motion and the motion that would be performed by the human body if it were subjected to the same controlling factors. The motions of the actual trial yielded nonconstant angular momentum values during free-fall, whereas the motions computed by the simulation were forced to yield constant angular momentum values. This discrepancy resulted in rotation errors. The major sources of error are attributed to the errors in the approximation of the inertia parameters of the segments and to the errors involved in the smoothing procedures.

INTERPRETATION OF TEST RESULTS

Limitations of the measurement techniques.   The analysis of the dynamics of human motion and body segment motions are usually performed by means of cinematography techniques and models. The most important sources of errors are introduced by the approximations regarding the segment characteristics such as masses, centers of mass, moments of inertia, and joint centers, and also by the approximations introduced in the smoothing and differentiation procedures. When all these errors are combined and are extended to the analysis of all body segments, they may lead to substantial fallacies with regard to the interpretation of the data. More research should be oriented toward the investigation of the relative effects of these errors upon both the kinematics and kinetics of human movement.

It is much easier to control the errors and specifically to know the degree of importance when techniques involving transducers are used. However, the type of information provided by these techniques is usually limited (ground reaction forces and force distribution under the foot), and these techniques must generally be combined with cinematography when more complete information is required.

Specificity of the results.   The time history of the moments of force at each joint gives valuable insight into the net effect of all agonist and antagonist muscles. These kinetic patterns may further be used to evaluate the power or the rate of work done by the muscle moments. The results on moments of force, however, do not provide specific information relative to the specific muscle forces and the process of co-contractions.

Modeling and the assumptions regarding the direction of muscular pulls and the sites of muscular attachment provide information about the action of specific muscles and the resulting joint reaction forces. This information is used to evaluate the specific requirements involved in a sport task and the risk factors associated with that task.

The measures of ground reaction forces and the pressure distribution give an insight into the patterns of impulse and the development of velocity attributed to these impulses generated on the external environment. However, these measurements are usually confined to one single support phase because of the limitations in the size of the force platforms. The pressure distribution is generally restricted to an axis normal to the platform. The pressure distribution allows the researcher to understand the areas of force concentration beneath the foot, and is mainly used to evaluate the characteristics of the support provided with different types of shoes.

The linear momentum may be measured during the contact and airborne phases of motion. The linear momentum is usually measured from force-time data (impulse) and is used to approximate the velocity development and the final velocity at takeoff. The final velocity of takeoff is used to predict some of the characteristics during the airborne phase such as the vertical displacement of the athlete and the horizontal displacement (in that case the time of flight must be known). The information about the angular momentum is of particular interest for activities such as jumping and diving; by simulation procedures the segmental contributions are examined in relation to their effects on the body orientation at any moment during the airborne phase.

Mechanical Energy, Work, and Efficiency

It is difficult to separate discussions of mechanical energy and work of human motion. The work done on a body segment or by the body taken as a whole is by definition the sum of the changes in energy level of the segment or of the total body center of gravity. That is, work must be done to change the amount of energy a body possesses. If the investigator can calculate the change in energy level, then the work done can also be calculated if the initial level is known. The athletic performance assessment is most practically used in calculating the work output. This calculation is accomplished by working from the knowledge of the changes in energy level, the so-called inverse dynamics problem. Mechanical efficiency is the ratio of the work output to metabolic cost. By itself this ratio is of little use in motion assessment; however, knowledge of both the mechanical and metabolic work rates is extremely valuable.

DEFINITIONS AND STANDARD UNITS

Energy (E) is the capacity to do work and exists in many forms including sound, electricity, heat, chemistry, and mechanics. In this discussion only mechanical energy is of direct interest, although heat equivalents must be used to relate mechanical to metabolic costs of a movement.

Mechanical energy has four forms: energy of position vertically above some defined reference level (potential energy, PE); energy of motion in straight lines (translatory kinetic energy, TKE); energy of motion in rotation (rotational kinetic energy, RKE); and energy of change in shape or configuration (strain or elastic energy). The first three forms can be readily calculated in many human movements but strain energy is not directly accounted for routinely.

$$PE = Wh \text{ or } Mgh \tag{3-19}$$

$$\text{TKE} = \frac{1}{2} Mv_G^2 \tag{3-20}$$

$$\text{RKE} = \frac{1}{2} I_{CM}\omega^2 \tag{3-21}$$

In the above equations, W = weight in Newtons (N); h = vertical distance or height above an arbitrarily defined reference level (datum) in meters (m); M = mass (kg); g = gravitational constant 9.81 m/s²; v = velocity of the center of mass (G) of the body or body segment (m/s); I = moment of inertia about center of mass (CM) in kg • m²; and ω = rotation (angular) velocity (rad/s).

The appropriate unit for PE, TKE, and RKE is the joule (J), which is equal to 1 N • m. The right sides of equations 3-19, 3-20, and 3-21 can all be reduced to N • m or J.

Mechanical work can be defined in two different ways, both of which are useful in human motion analyses.

The basic definition of Work (u) is that it is the product of a force (F) times the displacement (d) through which an object moves along the line of the force. If the force and the displacement are in the same direction the work is *positive*; if they are in opposite directions the work is *negative*. To lift a weight, for example, a force is applied to the weight in an upward direction and the weight moves up. To lower the weight the force is reduced in the upward direction and the weight moves down as a result of gravity but is under muscular control. Lifting the weight is positive work done by muscle on the weight; lowering the weight is negative work done by muscle to control the weight.

If the object is rotating, as human bodies or body segments often do, the work done is the product of the torque or moment of force (τ) times the angular displacement (θ; radians) with the same sense of positive or negative as for the linear case.

Work is also equal to the change in PE, TKE, and RKE levels because force (F), mass (M), acceleration (a), torque (τ), moment of inertia (I), and angular acceleration (α) are related. Moreover, acceleration, velocity, and displacement are also related for objects moving in straight lines or rotating.

The following set of equations demonstrates the above relationships:

$$u = F \cdot d \tag{3-22}$$

$$u = \tau \cdot \theta \tag{3-23}$$

$$u = \Delta TKE \text{ i.e. } \frac{1}{2} Mv^2_{CMf} - \frac{1}{2} Mv^2_{CMi} \qquad (3\text{-}24)$$

$$u = \Delta RKE \text{ i.e. } \frac{1}{2} I_{CM}\omega^2_f - \frac{1}{2} I_{CM}\omega^2_i \qquad (3\text{-}25)$$

$$u = \Delta PE \text{ i.e. } Mgh_f - Mgh_i \qquad (3\text{-}26)$$

where u = work done (N • m = J), F = force (N), d = linear displacement in meters (m), τ = moment of force or torque (N • m), θ = angular displacement (rad.), f and i indicate final and initial values, and Δ = change in; the remaining symbols were previously defined. The appropriate unit for work (u) as for energy (E) is the joule (J). 1 J = 1 N • m.

Mechanical efficiency is best defined as the ratio of the total work output to metabolic work output required to sustain this mechanical work. Total mechanical work output is comprised of the sum of the internal and external work (Cavagna & Kaneko, 1977; Winter, 1979b).

$$ME = \frac{\text{internal + external mechanical work} \times 100\%}{\text{metabolic work}} \qquad (3\text{-}27)$$

ME = mechanical efficiency. Internal and external mechanical work will be explained later.

A sizable divergence of opinion among biomechanists still exists as to how the mechanical work is most accurately calculated (cf. Williams & Cavanagh, 1983; Winter, 1979b) and among physiologists as to how the metabolic work is best represented (cf. Gaesser & Brooks, 1975). In general, the mechanical work in sport skills is usually calculated from film or some other form of imaging. The metabolic work is calculated from oxygen uptake measures. Both can be equated via known heat equivalents of mechanical work and liters of oxygen consumed, given certain assumptions about what type of substrate has been used metabolically.

LIMITATIONS

The information content of mechanical energy and work with regard to the analysis and assessment of athletic performance has not been fully exploited. The shapes and sizes of body segment energy curves and the phase relationships among the curves of several body segments are highly affected by the velocities of the segments, their relative masses, the motor coordination of the athlete, and the constraints of the movement itself. For example, the legs of a cyclist with toes locked in traps have a constrained movement pattern. The arm and leg movements of a cross-country skier, although constrained to some degree, can exhibit a larger variety of combinations.

In short, mechanical energy and work analyses are potentially very powerful analytical tools in sport. If the analysis is limited to movements of the total body center of gravity, the information yield will be low because the center of gravity analysis gives no direct information about the technique used by the athlete. The limbs are responsible for the center of gravity movements, and errors or problems with the pattern reside in the limbs in many cases. Therefore, body segment approaches are to be preferred.

Mechanical efficiency calculations, in which only the ratio of the mechanical work rate to metabolic rate is reported, are of limited, if any, use at all. The reason is that although a relationship exists between mechanical and metabolic costs of a movement in a heterogeneous range, highly skilled technique can compensate for relatively poor metabolic delivery system development, and vice versa. In relatively homogeneous groups knowledge of the mechanical work output, the mechanical energy curve changes that produced it, and the associated metabolic rates are important if the reasons for a particular mechanical efficiency are to be found.

A limitation of the mechanical work output methods is that they will not reflect improvements in muscular coordination that do not result in an overt body segment movement pattern change. In other words, if an athlete reduced unneeded muscular co-contractions one would say that skill was improved. But the resultant torque output could be the same even though it was produced by reduced agonist muscle activity. If so, then the movement of the body segment would not be changed. Skill was improved because the metabolic cost of performing that task was lower as a result of lower muscular activity. This example highlights the importance of knowing both the mechanical work output and the metabolic cost whenever possible to assess athletic performance.

Technically, the accuracy of the measurements depends on most of the factors identified as limitors in the muscular torque estimations. These include the accuracy of masses of the body segments, the validity of displacement data curve and smoothing, and numerical differentiation techniques employed. The filter cutoff frequency selected, for example, can have a large effect on the size of the total body work output calculated.

One advantage of a mechanical energy and work output approach over joint moment calculations is that joint moment calculations require the calculation of accelerations while mechanical energy and work output require only velocities. Errors in acceleration calculations are higher than in velocities. Furthermore, accurate joint movements require a force plate with its inherent constraints (see page 39). Work output is best calculated from the joint moment values (equation 3-23) but can be calculated from the body segment energy levels, albeit with somewhat less versatile interpretive value, from film data alone. So, work output is much more useful as a field site tool.

PURPOSE FOR MEASURING

These measurements are very detailed descriptors of movement patterns. Insofar as the movement pattern is a reflection of the skill of the athlete, the mechanical energy and work data reflect that skill also. If the athlete's technique can be improved, mechanical energy curves will show the change. The curves will permit localization to the particular body parts involved when there are overt movement pattern changes, that is, something visible to a camera, if not to the naked eye. If the detailed documentation of an athlete's technique is important, then these techniques are important to assessment of sport performance.

POTENTIAL USES FOR MEASUREMENT OF MOVEMENT PATTERNS

- Use measurements as baseline data on the current technique of junior and established athletes who are expected to improve.
- Compare movement patterns periodically with the baseline data as a follow-up to technique coaching and physiological conditioning (e.g., strength training) and to monitor the growth of juniors.
- Use movement patterns to document and assess the location on the body and the nature of technique breakdown as a result of fatigue during the course of an event.
- Compare the technique of one athlete with athletes considered to be more highly skilled.

RELEVANCE

Mechanical energy and work output measurements are potentially applicable to technique analysis and assessment of any movement pattern that contains measurable body segment velocities and vertical displacement changes. This type of analysis is not appropriate for static postures such as balance stunts in gymnastics.

The method proposed in chapter 5 is currently the most useful in analyzing movements that comply with the following criteria:

1. Essentially two dimensions (plane motion)
2. Cyclical (e.g., repetitive strides in running and cross-country skiing)
3. Result in overt body segment movement changes because of technique improvement, changes in strength or other physiological mechanisms, and fatigue onset (technique breakdown)

Table 3.2 is a list, though not exhaustive, of examples of sport or components of sport to which these techniques do and do not apply. Category I includes movements that can be analyzed very well via mechanical energy methods. Category II movements are usefully analyzed by these methods but with limitations because of third-dimension components or the fact that the movement is not cyclical. Category III shows a few examples in which this type of analysis is not useful because of the nature of the movement, or the analysis is currently very difficult because the movements are primarily in three dimensions. Mechanical efficiency can

Table 3.2 Work-Energy Applications to Sport

Category I[1]	Category II	Category III
Running—in any event Track Basketball Vaulting approaches in gymnastics	Vertical jumps Basketball Volleyball Diving approach	Airborne rotation Gymnastics Diving Figure skating
Walking—race walking	Plane motion rotations in gymnastics in continuous contact with apparatus (e.g., giant swings)	Ground contact twists or spins Figure skating Throwing events in track Baseball
Cross-country skiing Single or double poling Level or uphill	Straight line skating Hockey	Shooting in hockey
		Downhill skiing

[1]See text for explanation of categories.
I = highly relevant
II = somewhat relevant
III = not easily obtainable

be calculated only if both the total mechanical work output and metabolic cost can be usefully determined. It is not useful to calculate the
inefficiency of a single vertical jump, for example.

It should be noted that three-dimensional movement analysis techniques have been published (cf. Dapena, 1981), but they are not yet routinely done in most laboratories. Proposals for analysis of such movements
should be reviewed very critically to determine whether the author(s) has
the capability (e.g., debugged computer software) of doing this type of
work.

TESTING PROCEDURES

To introduce the testing procedures it is important to identify problems
that have emerged in the past with these types of calculations, then to
propose an approach that improves on work reported in this area in past
years. Mechanical energy, work, and efficiency are the topics of this section, and they are all closely related. The nature of the controversy is best
identified by concentrating on the issue of *mechanical efficiency*.

THE PROBLEM OF THE CONCEPT AND
CALCULATION OF MECHANICAL EFFICIENCY
OF ATHLETIC PERFORMANCE

The calculation of mechanical efficiency in various athletic movements
has been interesting for many years because of the assumed association
of such a numerical value with the skill of the performer. The term mechanical efficiency is frequently used to describe the amount of mechanical
work done as a proportion of the metabolic energy expended to do it
(equation 3-28). Moreover, an intuitive relationship exists between the
mechanical cost of a movement related to the athlete's technique and the
metabolic cost related to his or her physiological capacities. The technique
and the physiological parameters can be related in an attractive way because the units of measurement of both types of work can be equated.

$$\text{Efficiency} = \frac{\text{total mechanical work} \times 100\%}{\text{metabolic cost}} \qquad (3\text{-}28)$$

Two major problems are apparent, however: (a) What is the appropriate
numerical value that most accurately reflects the total mechanical work
in complex, multisegmental movement patterns such as running, bicycling, cross-country skiing, swimming, and so on and (b) What is the best
measure of the metabolic cost, particularly when the movement has an
appreciable anaerobic component?

The total mechanical work output is the sum of the internal and external work (equation 3-27, page 48). The external work is usually easy to measure directly from the scale on a bicycle ergometer, the amount of weight lifted, or the size of a pushed, pulled, or carried load. If no external load is involved, as in walking or running, then this external work has been calculated simply from the total rise (or lowering in downhill locomotion) of the center of gravity of the body such as in inclined treadmill running (e.g., Margaria, 1968). Of course, in level locomotion no net raising or lowering of the total body center of gravity occurs. The external work output is zero, but the metabolic cost is not zero. The efficiency of such forms of locomotion is calculated to be zero, clearly an anomalous value.

To handle this problem Cavagna, Saibene, and Margaria (1964) defined *external work* as that fraction of the total mechanical work necessary to sustain the displacements of the center of gravity. They calculated this value from the changes in horizontal kinetic energy and potential energy (vertical displacements) of the total body center of gravity.

Cavagna et al. (1964) calculated the *internal mechanical work* from the movements of the limbs relative to the total body center of gravity using a technique proposed by Fenn (1930). The internal work was defined as

> that fraction (of the total) that does not lead to a displacement of the centre of gravity of the system and which is required a) to overcome muscle viscosity and joint friction, b) to sustain isometric contractions and c) those movements of the limbs which do not lead to a displacement of the centre of gravity. Only component c) can be measured through an analysis of the limb movements. (p. 249)

In this definition, there seems to be a mixing of mechanical work sources and metabolic energy consumers. Friction and isometric muscular contractions perform no mechanical work but are metabolic energy consumers. Furthermore, Smith (1975a) has convincingly pointed out some unjustified assumptions in the Fenn (1930) and consequently in the Cavagna et al. (1964) calculations. In addition, this approach seems to discount the fact that the limb movements are the cause of the motion of the center of gravity and are not extraneous to it. In this respect the work done to produce motion of the limbs should be included in any calculation of mechanical efficiency.

Notwithstanding these criticisms of the methods of calculating and separating internal and external work, Cavagna and his colleagues have clearly demonstrated the importance of including limb movements in the measurement of total work output. Although internal mechanical work is not as easy to measure as external work, Cavagna and Kaneko (1977) have shown that internal work amounts to more than the external work of walking at all speeds and in running at speeds greater than 20 km/hr.

Even in bicycle ergometry, a task where trunk movements are of low velocity and low vertical displacement change compared with running or walking, Kaneko and Yamazaki (1978) have shown that the amounts of internal work were 7% to 27% of the external work. For the above reasons the best representation of efficiency is equation 3-27 (page 48).

To further complicate the matter, not only is the question of whether it is necessary to include a measure of internal work in the efficiency calculation at issue, to say nothing of how to calculate it, but so is the appropriate number for the metabolic cost. We do not plan to handle this matter here because it is a physiological rather than biomechanical problem. However, a paragraph is appropriate to delineate the options.

Gaesser and Brooks (1975) compared traditional and theoretical exercise efficiency calculations during steady-rate cycle ergometer exercises at various work rates and velocities. They calculated muscular efficiencies in four ways by changing the metabolic work rate components. Interestingly, they paid no attention at all to the equally perplexing problem of the appropriate method of calculating the mechanical work. Their gross efficiency employed the measurement of gross oxygen cost, net efficiency used the measurement of the metabolic energy expended above that in cycling with zero load, and delta efficiency used the change in mechanical work accomplished with a new load or velocity divided by the corresponding change in oxygen cost.

The delta efficiency proved to decline both with increases in work rate and velocity, but the net and gross efficiencies increased unexpectedly with increases in work rate but declined with increases in velocity. On this basis Gaesser and Brooks seemed to promote the delta efficiency, although it is not clear why an increase in work rate should necessarily produce a reduction in efficiency.

The long and short of the entire problem of calculating a single number called efficiency (supposedly indicative of the quality of human movement) is that the magnitude of that number depends on exactly what the author chose to include in the calculation of both the mechanical work output and metabolic cost. Mainly as a result of differences in methods of calculation of efficiency rather than differences in performance, a review of the literature reveals disparate values for the reasonably common task of running, which range from about 25% (Margaria, Cerretelli, & Sassi, 1963) to 70% or 80% (Cavagna & Kaneko, 1977), excluding Margaria's value of 0% for level running (Margaria, 1968).

Some standardization of approach is obviously required if the quality of human performance is to be usefully assessed in this way. In fact, it appears unrealistic to hope for a single index of human performance. For example, Norman, Sharratt, Pezzack, and Noble (1976), in a study of efficiency of treadmill running of a small homogeneous group, suggested that it is desirable for a runner to run at a given velocity at a low mechanical work output and at low metabolic cost. Equations 3-27 and 3-28 (pages 48 and 52), however, indicate that a high efficiency calculation results from a high mechanical work output at low metabolic cost. One of the runners exhibited such a combination. The other two runners could run at the same velocity with lower mechanical work output but higher metabolic cost. Thus their technique efficiency seemed relatively good and their metabolic efficiency apparently was not as good.

To make the best use of this type of information, knowledge of both the mechanical work output and metabolic cost is necessary. In addition, both the internal and external mechanical work output must be measured along with individual body segment energy level changes if diagnosis of technique is to be possible from these mechanical efficiency measures.

INTERPRETATION OF TEST RESULTS

Some comments concerning specificity of these measurements can be found on page 48 under Limitations. Further inference as to specificity in the sense of applicability to particular sports can be made by reviewing pages 50-52, Relevance.

There are limitations to this measurement technique:

1. Measurements of mechanical work output from assumed potential energy changes of the total body center of gravity during inclined treadmill running (e.g., Margaria, 1968) are of very little value and are, indeed, erroneous. This technique cannot be used at all for movements on a level surface because no net rise exists in the center of gravity.
2. Measurements of external work rate from the scale on a bicycle ergometer are underestimations by about 7% to 27% for work loads of 5 to 1 kp, respectively, according to Kaneko and Yamazaki (1978). Subtracting metabolic rate at unloaded pedaling from that obtained with a load yields an apparent mechanical efficiency value of about 26%, which is in line with the efficiencies calculated by including both the internal and external mechanical work rate and dividing simply by the corresponding metabolic rate.

   However, if sources of possible inefficiencies in competitive cycling were of interest, it would be imperative to calculate both the internal and external work, the internal work from an analysis of the moving limbs.
3. A rough estimate of the total body energy curves and corresponding work output can be calculated from the vertical displacement and velocity changes of the total body center of gravity. These data can be obtained from film analysis or other imaging techniques or from

force plate or accelerometer records (e.g., Cavagna & Margaria, 1966; Cavagna, Komarck, & Mazzoleni, 1971).

The time history of changes in these energy patterns can be observed and the potential and kinetic energy components can be separated. The interaction of these two components provides some indication of the skill of the performer, that is, the relative degree of vertical oscillations in displacement versus horizontal velocity changes, and places the oscillations and changes on a comparable scale. However, just as much diagnostic information might be found in the displacement and velocity data themselves. Furthermore, Winter (1979b) has shown that these center of gravity measures underestimate the total body work output from linked segment analyses of walking by an average of 16%, with some differences as high as 42%. The main reason is that the work done by oscillating limbs is not accounted for if it does not lead to changes in the location or velocity of the center of gravity.

Even when properly derived, analysis of the total body energy curves gives very little information about how the athlete used his or her body segments to produce the total body movement pattern. Consequently, if a project proposes to produce only the total body energy curves based on total body center of gravity measurements, the information content would be extremely limited.

4. The linked segment approach to mechanical energy, work output, and mechanical efficiency is preferred. The segment energy level changes provide important information about the athlete's ability to effectively coordinate the independent and interdependent movements of the limbs. The total body work output and an estimate of work done in the body segments individually can be obtained.

However, this approach, too, has its limitations. If the work output is obtained from the analysis of body segment energies, then the actual work done by the muscles crossing the joints (the variable ultimately of interest) is obtained only by inference. This inference becomes very uncertain when transfers of energy from one segment to another are of interest, particularly when the segments are not adjacent but are attached by multijoint muscles (cf. Williams & Cavanagh, 1983).

A more direct approach to muscle work output, therefore, is via the joint torque (moment of force): angular displacement method (equation 3-23, page 47). But while this technique is mechanically more accurate than that of the segment energy, it suffers from all of the limitations of the joint torque calculation, the requirement of the use of a force plate, and its accompanying restrictions. Force plates, of course, are usually impractical for obtaining data during cyclical competitive events (e.g., several running striders), and have other constraints, noted earlier.

Linked-segment mechanical work analysis as proposed in chapter 5 does not separate internal and external work. A load on the back, for example, is considered simply another segment in the linkage or an increase in trunk mass. Although some may consider this a limitation, this type of analysis is coherent and biomechanically and physiologically sound. As noted by Winter (1979b), linked-segment mechanical work analysis accounts for the following:

- Three of four energy components, potential and translatory and rotational kinetic energy. It does not account for stored elastic energy (see Cavagna, 1977 for a review of elasticity). This would appear, however, in a lowered metabolic rate for a given mechanical work rate.
- All energy exchanges known to occur both among body segments and between potential and kinetic energy within segments.
- Positive and negative work.

Furthermore, linked-segment mechanical work analysis permits an analysis of the mechanical energy changes in various body segments, the segment movement patterns being undoubtedly reflections of the sources of mechanical or technique inefficiencies.

4

Neuromuscular Considerations

PIERRE LAGASSE

The technique of electromyography (EMG) is used to study the electrical activity produced by a muscle during its contraction. Because human movements originate from contractions of various muscles of the body that orchestrate their individual actions to produce efficient movement, the actual amount of electricity generated by these muscles has been studied for many years. Electromyography is a research tool commonly used to study daily life movements and athletic movements in symptomatic and asymptomatic human beings. It is, however, a complex technique that requires sophisticated hardware. The electromyogram in itself is a complex signal that can be influenced at any given time by many variables and whose interpretation is even more complex (Figure 4.1). Therefore, the

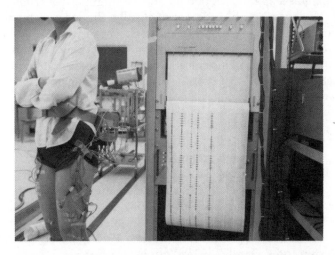

Figure 4.1 EMG recording systems: 16 channel telemetry transmitter, electrodes on several leg muscles and unprocessed records on recorder.

following section will focus primarily on EMG parameters that have previously been shown to be valid and reliable measures, and that have been demonstrated to be pertinent indicators of human athletic ability.

Definition and Explanation of the Parameters

One of the characteristics of skilled performance is that the muscles responsible for the execution of movement exhibit a specific sequential and temporal order of activation. Several authors (Finley, Wirta, & Cody, 1967; Gatev, 1972; Hobart, Kelley, & Bradley, 1975; Hobart & Vorro, 1974; Hobart, Vorro, & Dotson, 1978; Kamon & Gormley, 1968; Komarek, 1968; Normand, Lagasse, Rouillard, & Tremblay, 1982; Payton & Kelley, 1972; Person, 1958; Vorro, 1973; Vorro & Hobart, 1974; Vorro & Hobart, 1981a, b) have demonstrated that the acquisition of a novel motor task involves using the neuromuscular system to transform the sequential and temporal order of activation of the various agonist, antagonist, and synergist muscles involved in the execution of the task. Researchers generally believe that sustained practice of a motor task establishes an advanced level of muscular control and economy of effort. Thus the muscles involved in the execution of the task exhibit an earlier premovement contraction and require less time to reach peak activity (Vorro & Hobart, 1981a).

The temporal and sequential order of muscle activation can be defined as the numerical and temporal order by which the first action potential reaches the motor point of the principal agonist, antagonist, and synergist muscles that are solicited for the execution of a movement. Because elite athletes exhibit a specific sequential and temporal order of muscle activation in the execution of their specific skills, the measurement of this parameter should be of great interest to coaches as a good indicator of the level of skill reached by lower caliber athletes. The measurement may also enlighten the desired modifications in sequential and temporal order of muscle activation that could produce further improvement in performance.

REACTION TIME

Reaction time of athletes has been shown to be substantially faster than reaction time of nonathletes (Kroll & Clarkson, 1978). This faster reaction time has been demonstrated for varsity athletes (Olsen, 1956; Slater-Hammel, 1955), for fencers (Pierson, 1956), for top racquetball players (Knapp, 1961). Several studies have also shown that athletes of different sports have different reaction times (Burley, 1944; Cureton, 1951; Keller, 1942; Westerlund & Tuttle, 1931; Youngen, 1959).

An important question is, What makes athletes react faster to external stimuli? Is a faster reaction time due to faster central nervous system processing, rapid nerve conduction velocity, or faster speeds of muscle contraction? Kroll and Clarkson (1978) reviewed several studies (Kato, 1960; Street, 1968) that have demonstrated that athletes of different disciplines have similar nerve conduction velocities, and they do not differ from nonathletes on this parameter. Kato (1960) suggested that fast reaction times of athletes may be attributed to the superior functioning of the central nervous system. Kato's hypothesis was verified by Mosely (1974) and by Bodine-Reese and Bone (1976), who demonstrated that women athletes have faster premotor times than nonathletes. The data suggest that the faster reaction speeds may be the result of a faster central processing in the athletes.

Fractionated reaction time refers to the partitioning of total reaction time into premotor and motor time components. Premotor time is the interval of time between the presentation of the stimulus and the appearance of the first action potential recorded from the voluntarily reacting muscle group. Motor time is the period of time between the appearance of the first recorded muscle action potential and the beginning of movement. Because athletes do exhibit faster reaction times, the fractionation technique allows the researcher to identify the site (central or peripheral) responsible for this enhanced response. Furthermore, the technique can be used to specifically help identify the causes for slower reaction times in lower caliber athletes.

Involuntary responses, better known as reflexes, have been reported to be faster in athletes such as sprinters and middle-distance runners, and long-distance runners (Lautenbach & Tuttle, 1932). As with reaction time, total reflex time can be fractionated into nervous system and motor system components (Hayes, 1972). For example, by recording the time between a patellar tendon tap and the arrival of an efferent nerve impulse at the motor point, the traditional reflex latency can be secured (Kroll & Morris, 1976). Furthermore, because the total reflex time corresponds to the time between the tendon tap and the initial movement of the heel off a microswitch, the researcher can secure reflex motor time by simply subtracting the reflex latency from the total reflex time.

FIBER TYPE

Muscles of weight-trained athletes have been shown to have a greater percentage composition of fast-twitch fibers when compared to the average population (Costill et al., 1976; Edstrom & Ekblom, 1972; Gollnick, Armstrong, Saubert, Piehl, & Saltin, 1972) and that endurance athletes possess a greater percentage of slow-twitch muscle fibers (Costill et al.,

1976; Gollnick et al., 1972). Not only are the properties of the muscle different between power-trained and endurance-trained athletes, but a difference may also exist in the manner in which these fibers are used or recruited. Stepanov and Burlakov (1961) examined the EMG firing patterns in weight lifters and endurance athletes. They reported that endurance athletes demonstrated firing patterns that were asynchronous whereas weight lifters had a synchronous pattern where motor units are recruited in a simultaneous fashion. Such fiber characteristics and recruitment abilities make sense for the type of activities specific to power and endurance events. For power athletes, having a greater percentage of fast-twitch fibers would be advantageous due to the fibers' ability to generate tension and contract quickly. For endurance athletes, having a greater percentage of slow-twitch fibers would be advantageous due to the slow-twitch fibers' ability to resist fatigue and to fire asynchronously, assuring rest of some fibers while others are active.

The ability to rapidly contract a muscle, called muscular power, can be monitored by time to peak tension curves. In this particular test, an athlete is asked to achieve maximal voluntary contraction in a minimal amount of time. Furthermore, by monitoring the EMG activity of the contracting muscle, the investigator can assess the electromechanical delay (Norman & Komi, 1979), which is the time elapsed between the appearance on the EMG record of the first action potential at the motor point of the contracting muscle and the beginning of the rise in the tension curve. Hypothetically, power athletes should reach maximal voluntary tension faster than endurance athletes, and their electromechanical delay should be shorter. Recent data indicate that time to peak tension curves and electromechanical delays are good predictors of performance for power events (Lagasse, Dion, Rouillard, & Normand, 1981).

Purpose for Measuring the Different Neuromuscular Parameters and Their Relevance

The purpose for measuring neuromuscular parameters in athletes is to assess the modifications that occur during the process of skill acquisition in the neuromuscular system as a result of training. Because all of the neuromuscular parameters presented in the previous section have been shown to be modifiable by training and to exhibit specific characteristics in athletes, their measurement can be very relevant to the skill or proficiency level attained by these athletes.

The temporal and sequential order of muscle activation has been shown to be modified by practice. Champion athletes demonstrate a specific temporal and sequential order of muscle activation in the execution of their specific skill. Modifications that occur in this parameter as a result of practice are attributable to a reorganization in the central nervous system of the motor program required to execute a specific task. Several studies have demonstrated that modifications in the central nervous system motor program manifest themselves by inhibiting the undesired activity from the antagonist muscles (Gatev, 1972; Kamon & Gormley, 1968; Komarek, 1968; Normand et al., 1982). Therefore, the measurement of this parameter can be relevant to determining the level of proficiency attained by an athlete and can enlighten the desired modifications in sequential and temporal order of muscle activation, which can produce further improvement in performance.

Both reaction and reflex times have a long history of study due to their inherent qualities as simple indicators of the status of the neuromuscular system. The importance of reaction time in the study of human athletic performance is well established, especially in athletic skills that require a reaction from the performer to a specific stimulus. Furthermore, few sports exist in which reaction time is not important. In basketball, for example, the ability to start and stop instantly with sudden changes in direction is an indispensable characteristic. No coach would deny that the capacity to react quickly with agility and coordination is one of the most important factors of athletic performance.

The significance of muscle reflexes, however, is less apparent until one recognizes that reflexes are capable of facilitatory or inhibitory influences upon volitional muscle action (Fukuda, 1961). Muscle reflexes have been implicated in developmental patterns of physical skill acquisition (Connolly, 1970). In fact, some authors have suggested that the muscle reflex is a basic element in all skilled motor behavior (Gottlieb & Agarwal, 1972) and that muscle reflexes underlie most of man's volitional movements (Easton, 1972), representing a basic building block of motor coordination and skilled performance. Even though the importance of reflex time in the study of human athletic performance has not been as well established as it has been for reaction time, several studies have demonstrated that athletes subjected to various training regimens exhibit faster reflex times (Francis & Tipton, 1969; Reid, 1967; Tipton & Karpovich, 1966). It seems that reflex times are as important as reaction times in human athletic performance.

Using a technique to fractionate reaction and reflex times into nervous system and muscle contraction latencies offers additional and more substantive information than traditional unfractionated reaction and reflex time techniques. Total reaction time can be fractionated into premotor time and motor time components corresponding to central processing and motor output functions (Kroll & Clarkson, 1978). Likewise, total reflex time can be fractionated into reflex latency and motor time components with a similar correspondence to central and peripheral components (Kroll

& Clarkson, 1978). Identification of the locus and magnitude of changes in reaction and reflex time for athletes of different skill levels may illuminate the mechanisms involved in both skilled and unskilled performance. An added benefit can be obtained by securing both fractionated reflex and fractionated reaction times. Because total reaction time is comprised of a volitional central nervous system component (for example, premotor time) while total reflex time is comprised of a nonvolitional central nervous system component (for example, the reflex latency), information is provided about volitional versus nonvolitional changes in the central nervous system. These changes are reflected in the premotor time and the reflex latency components and in the muscular contractions produced by volitional versus nonvolitional nervous system control (Kroll & Clarkson, 1978).

The ability to rapidly contract a muscle and reach a desired level of muscular tension represents a neuromuscular quality that appears to be important in athletic performance, especially in power events. Even though an athlete may have a fast reaction time to an external stimulus, his ability to rapidly contract a muscle and reach a desired level of muscle tension may not necessarily be fast because the rate of tension development of human muscles is known to be related to the percent distribution of fast-twitch fibers (Viitasalo & Komi, 1981). The rate of tension development is also related to the firing patterns of the motor units that are recruited (Stepanov & Burlakov, 1961), whereas reaction time depends largely on central nervous system processing time such as premotor time. No doubt, athletes and coaches will agree that muscle strength is an important part of athletic ability, especially in power events. They will also agree that muscle tension is important not only in terms of the quantity of muscular tension developed but also in terms of the time required for the development of this tension.

The four neuromuscular parameters presented probably could be measured on all types of athletes. It seems particularly important to measure the sequential and temporal order of muscle activation on fine motor skill athletes such as basketball players, volleyball players, and racquet sport players and to assess rate of tension development capacity on all power athletes.

Testing Procedures

The testing procedures and measurement techniques that are currently being used to assess the sequential and temporal order of muscle activation, fractionated reaction time, fractionated reflex time, and rate of tension development have been very well standardized over the years and have gained universal recognition. To attempt to compare various measurement techniques or tests used for strengths and weaknesses would be useless and impossible. This section will simply attempt to describe as accurately as possible the usual procedure used to measure the neuromuscular parameters.

To assess the temporal and sequential order of muscle activation for a specific sport, the researcher must first identify a particular movement of interest for that sport. For example, a volleyball coach may have a special interest in the spike movement of his or her athletes. The specific joints that play an important part in the execution of this skill must also be identified. The shoulder and elbow joints, for example, are particularly active in the volleyball spike. For each joint, one agonist muscle and its antagonist must be selected. Because the technique that will be proposed for the measurement of this parameter is surface electromyography, the muscles selected must be accessible for study by this technique, so they must be superficial muscles. For the study of the volleyball spike, the pectoralis major and the posterior deltoid could be the musles selected for EMG study of the shoulder joint, and the biceps and triceps brachii muscles could be the muscles selected for the EMG study of the elbow joint. Furthermore, because the electromyographical records obtained from each muscle must be related to the movement studied, using a measurement device to monitor segment position is also convenient. Because its signal can be recorded on the same apparatus as EMG signals, thereby eliminating synchronization problems, an electrogoniometer or an accelerometer can record segment position and displacement.

Surface electromyography as it is used to assess sequential and temporal order of muscle activation parameters has been shown to be a valid technique, as long as the possible sources of errors that are associated with this technique (see chapter 5) are well controlled by the experimenter. The reliability of the various measurements that this technique yields, (e.g., motor times, activity times, and latency times) is well beyond acceptable (R > .80) levels (Lagasse, 1979). Perhaps the major source of error associated with this technique is the technique of electrogoniometry recommended to monitor segment position and displacement. Because human segmental movements are rarely biaxial and most commercially available electrogoniometers or accelerometers monitor only biaxial movement, errors can result. This weakness, however, can be eliminated by using triaxial accelerometers or electrogoniometers to monitor body segment position and displacement.

To assess fractionated reaction times for athletes of a specific sport, first determining which muscle group is particularly responsible for initiating the fast reactions that are specific to that sport is important. For example, plantar flexors of the foot are more important for sprinters than are forearm flexors. Again, because the technique for determining fractionated reaction time components (see chapter 5) is electromyography, the selected muscle must be superficial. The type of stimulus (visual vs. auditory) most appropriate for a specific sport should also be determined, because reaction time to an auditory stimulus is faster than reaction time to a visual stimulus. The technique that is used to assess reaction time should attempt to eliminate subject anticipation to presentation of the stimulus. This problem can be remedied by randomly varying the time elapsed between the preparatory signal and the actual presentation of the stimulus. Furthermore, because reaction times have been shown to improve with practice the experimental design should incorporate a practice session, for example, between 20 and 50 practice trials, prior to the actual testing.

Using the EMG technique to fractionate reaction time into premotor and motor time components is valid as long as the possible sources of error are controlled. Premotor time, motor time, and total reaction time are stable measures and their reliability coefficients can be expected to be around .90.

Determining which muscle group contributes most to movement execution is important when assessing fractionated reflex time for athletes of a specific sport. The muscle that is selected for fractionated reflex time determination should be superficial because electromyography is used to fractionate this parameter into its nervous system and peripheral components. The subject's anticipation to the tendon tap stimulus, which would tend to influence the electromyographic record, can be eliminated by blindfolding him or her. With well controlled sources of error the assessment of fractionated reflex times with surface electromyography is a valid technique. The reliability of total reflex time and reflex motor time is high ($R > .85$). The reliability of reflex latency is relatively low ($R \simeq .60$), but this low reliability coefficient is attributable to low true score variance (for example, not much variation between subjects) and not to measurement instability.

The determination of rate of tension development and of the associated electromechanical delay requires the use of dynamometry and electromyography. The muscle group that is responsible for attaining a desired tension level for a particular sport should be carefully identified. Again, this muscle should be superficial because surface electromyography will be the recommended technique (see chapter 5) to assess the electromechanical delay. A force transducer is used to monitor the muscle tension generated by the contracting muscle. For synchronization purposes, recording the muscle tension signal on the same apparatus that is used for EMG recording is preferable.

As pointed out by Kamen (1980), the methodology used for the analysis of the force-time curve is quite varied. In 1964, Clarke advocated the usage of exponential curve-fitting techniques to quantify time-duration curves and reported a correlation of $-.79$ between the time to reach an arbitrary force measure and maximal handgrip strength. However, Clarke's single exponent rate constant failed to correlate with maximal voluntary contraction ($r \simeq -.03$). Willems (1973) adopted another procedure that consisted of computing the angle formed by the tangent to the force-time curve and the horizontal at the point corresponding to 50% and 90% of maximal isometric tension. A third procedure suggested by other investigators (Soderberg, 1977; Stothart, 1973) consists of computing such measures as the time to production of peak force and the maximal rate of tension development.

The technique proposed by Kamen (1980) will be used to describe the force-time characteristics of a maximal isometric contraction performed as rapidly as possible. The technique involves the computation of the following variables:

F_{1000} = force reached in 1000 ms.

$Slope_{max}$ = highest value for rate of tension development attained in 1000 ms.

$T\text{-}Slope_{max}$ = the time required to reach the highest value for rate of tension development.

$T_{1/2}$ = time to attain 50% of F_{1000}.

Reliability for electromechanical delay can be expected to be high ($R \simeq .90$) because this parameter is as stable as the motor time associated with total reaction time. Stability for the variables selected to describe the force-time curve characteristics can also be expected to be high ($R \simeq .90$) except for the time to reach the maximum rate of tension development ($R \simeq .65$) (Kamen, 1980).

Interpretation of Test Results

An example of an electromyographic record taken to measure the sequential and temporal order of muscle activation is presented in Figure 4.2 (Normand et al., 1982). This record was taken on a subject executing a maximal speed arm adduction movement immediately followed by a maximal speed forearm flexion. It shows the electromyographical activity of the pectoralis major, posterior deltoid, biceps brachii, and triceps brachii as well as the displacement curves of the arm and forearm segments. PMMT and BBMT refer to the motor times: for example, the time elapsed between the appearance of the first action potential at the motor point of the muscles tested and the onset of movement of the pectoralis major and biceps brachii muscles. PDAT and TBAT refer to the total activity time of the posterior deltoid and triceps brachii muscles, whereas PDTL and

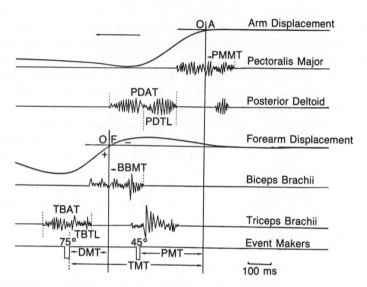

Figure 4.2 Sequential and Temporal Order of Muscle Activation. From "Modifications Occurring in Motor Programs During Learning of a Complex Task in Man" by M.C. Normand, P.P. Lagasse, C.A. Rouillard, and L.E. Tremblay, 1982, *Brain Research*. Copyright 1982 by Normand. Reprinted by permission.

TBTL represent the time between the onset of EMG activity and the end of the movement for the posterior deltoid and triceps brachii muscles.

The interpretation of an electromyographic record to assess the sequential and temporal order of muscle activation should focus (a) on the overlap of agonist and antagonist muscle activity and (b) on the onset of antagonist muscle activity prior to the end of movement because these two characteristics have been shown to be modifiable by practice or skill acquisition. For example, in a skilled athlete, agonist muscle activity (see Figure 4.2, EMG of pectoralis major and biceps brachii) ceases before onset of EMG activity in the antagonist muscle and no overlap of activity occurs between these two muscles. Furthermore, in skilled athletes the onset of antagonist muscle activity in relation to the end of movement (see Figure 4.2, PDTL and TBTL) can be expected to be shorter. Thus skilled athletes need less time to stop the ongoing movement of the limb by the action of the antagonist muscles.

An example of an electromyographical record taken to assess fractionated reaction times is presented in Figure 4.3. This record was taken on a subject reacting to a visual stimulus by adducting his horizontally suspended arm as soon as possible after appearance of the stimulus (Fleury & Lagasse, 1979). The record shows the electromyographical activity of

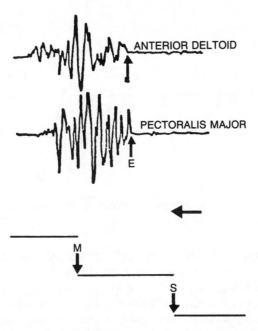

Figure 4.3 EMG and Fractionated Reaction Time. From "Influence of Functional Electrical Stimulation Training on Premotor and Motor Reaction Time" by M. Fleury and P. Lagasse, 1979, *Perceptual and Motor Skills*, **48**, pp. 387–393. Copyright 1979 by Fleury & Lagasse. Reprinted by permission.

the anterior deltoid and pectoralis major, two of the agonist muscles responsible for the adduction of the horizontally suspended arm. S represents the appearance of the visual stimulus, E corresponds to onset of electromyographic activity, and M corresponds to the onset of movement. Total reaction time is the time elapsed between points S and M, premotor time corresponds to the time between points S and E, and motor time is represented by the time difference between points E and M. Total reaction times of 210 ms, premotor times of 125 ms, and motor times of 85 ms are considered fast. Therefore, an athlete with a total reaction of 250 ms is considered slow-reacting. One of the advantages of fractionating total reaction time into its premotor and motor times components is that it permits the researcher to identify the locus and magnitude of changes in reaction and may serve to illuminate the mechanisms (central vs. peripheral) responsible for longer reactions. This type of information can be advantageously used to select appropriate training techniques.

An example of an electromyographical record taken from a storage oscilloscope to assess fractionated reflex time is presented in Figure 4.4. The reflex elicited is a patellar tendon reflex. Point T on the figure represents

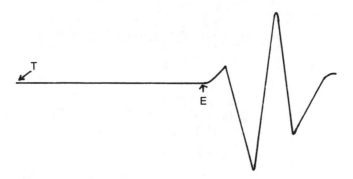

Figure 4.4 Oscillographic Record of Synchronized EMG.

the moment when the hammer made contact with the tendon, and point E represents the onset of muscle activity. Reflex latency is the time elapsed between the tendon tap and the appearance of the first action potential at the motor point of the stimulated muscle. Total reflex time can be obtained by using a clock that measures the interval between the tendon tap and onset of movement, whereas reflex motor time is obtained by subtracting reflex latency from total reflex time. For a normal population, patellar tendon reflex time is around 110 ms, with reflex latencies of 20 ms and reflex motor times of 90 ms. for power athletes, these values are 90, 20, and 70 ms, whereas they are 105, 20, and 85 ms for endurance athletes (Kroll & Clarkson, 1978). Fractionating total reflex time into its nervous system and peripheral components is advantageous, and the information that the total reflex time yields can be used to select appropriate training techniques.

An example of a dynamometry and electromyography record to assess rate of tension development and its associated electromechanical delay is presented in Figure 4.5. The maximal voluntary contraction studied is an isometric knee extension. Point E on the figure represents the onset of muscle activity in the vastus lateralis, and point T represents the beginning of the rise of the tension curve. The electromechanical delay is the time elapsed between points E and T. F_{1000} is the force reached 1000 ms after point T and $T_{1/2}$ represents the time needed to attain 50% of F_{1000}. Interpretation of the rate of tension development curves should consider the type of athletes, for example, power-trained versus endurance-trained athletes. Power-trained athletes are expected to have the ability to generate more tension in less time than endurance-trained athletes, and power-trained athletes' electromechanical delay should be shorter because of the specific type of their muscle fibers. Therefore, interpretation of these

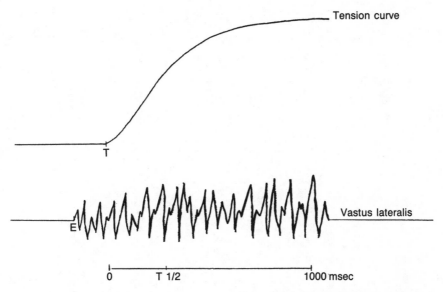

Figure 4.5 Rate of Tension Development Showing Electromechanical Delay.

results should be based on comparisons between athletes of the same and of different categories in order to properly assess their significance. For example, a power athlete that could develop tension at a slower rate than endurance-trained athletes should be prescribed a muscle power training program to improve his or her rate of tension development.

5

Recommended Procedures

DAVID DAINTY
MICHELINE GAGNON
PIERRE LAGASSE
ROBERT NORMAN
GORDON ROBERTSON
ERIC SPRIGINGS

Technique is discussed extensively in this chapter: how to perform certain tests, what problems to be wary of, and what equipment to use. Due to the nature of biomechanics, it is difficult to be all-inclusive in defining and describing test protocols. However, a number of methodologies are presented in this chapter, ranging from filming techniques to how to determine actual biomechanical parameters such as intersegmental energy transfers and ground reaction forces.

The necessary equipment is presented in most cases. One piece of equipment that is not discussed in any detail but is of great importance in any type of biomechanical test situation is the computer, whether a mainframe, mini, or microcomputer, and the necessary peripherals. A good and appropriate computing system has become a necessity to ensure rapid turnover of information and permit a sufficient number of subjects to be tested and their results to be analyzed (Figure 5.1). On-line testing facilities with sophisticated graphic outputs have become an everyday necessity in many good biomechanics laboratories. Although testing and analyses can be performed by hand, the capabilities afforded the investigator by a good computer system enhance the interpretation and presentation of results. Therefore, although computing systems are not discussed, they should be considered an integral part of any test situation.

The chapter is divided into a number of sections, each handling the different testing procedures presented in the preceding chapters. Each

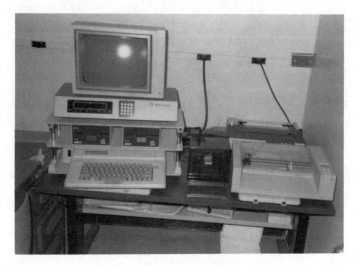

Figure 5.1   Microcomputer system for data acquisition, reduction, and analysis.

one of these procedures is discussed under the following subheadings: (a) actual protocol, (b) equipment specifications, (c) calibration procedures and expected reliability, and (d) other considerations. In a number of places, references are cited for specific topics. Please refer to the list of references for further information.

The use and availability of much of the equipment and technology presented is limited in many cases to university or private laboratories employing a number of specialists including biomechanists, computer technicians, laboratory technicians, and possibly graduate students. Utilizing these experts and facilities requires a certain level of funding. To give an example of the expected costs, a typical testing situation using a cinematographical approach is given in Appendix D. The costs are only a guideline and may be higher or lower depending on the facility and the personnel contracted. The contractor must carefully consider the expertise of those contracted and remember that although many test situations can be performed relatively cheaply, the information obtained may not be useful to anyone.

Cinematography

Regardless of whether a two-dimensional (2-D) or three-dimensional (3-D) approach is undertaken, the researcher must first select an experimentally verified filming technique from the literature and then follow the procedure accurately.

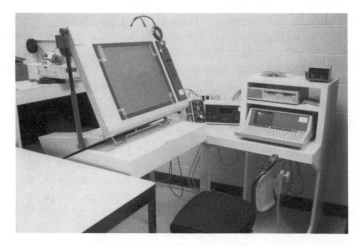

Figure 5.2 Back projection and computer interfaced film analyzer.

2-D CINEMATOGRAPHY

The 2-D filming procedure outlined in Miller and Nelson (1973) should be followed.

Equipment Specifications. Motor-driven cameras are best because they will assure the researcher a more constant time interval between frames. Spring-driven cameras may be used for qualitative research, but their limited accuracy would prohibit their use in most quantitative studies.

High quality camera lenses should be used to reduce lens distortion of the film image. A good quality zoom lens will prove most valuable to the researcher because this will allow a maximum image size.

A good quality film analyzer and digitizer are important for the quantification of film data points. A quality analyzer should provide film magnification in excess of 25 times the film size and should pin register each frame precisely in the gate for consistent analysis. A good digitizer should provide a resolution in the range of 0.1 mm to 0.5 mm (Figure 5.2).

Calibration Procedures and Expected Reliability. The true filming rate should be measured from information gathered during the actual filming sequence. This rate may be achieved by reading the values recorded on a digital or analog clock located in the field of view of each frame of film. It may also be achieved by counting the recorded pulses/s left on the film by an internal timing light. The researcher is discouraged from using indirect filming rate measurement methods such as (a) dropping an object in the photographic plane, (b) filming a running clock before or after the actual filming sequence, or (c) using the filming rate set on the control dial of the camera without having ascertained its validity beforehand.

With regard to accurately computing the scaling factor, the object of known length that is placed in the photographic plane must be of sufficient length to nullify the digitization errors of the two end points. Most operators can probably digitize to an accuracy no greater than 0.2 mm on the screen. Thus the sufficient length of the image of the known object would have to be at least 8 cm in order to keep the maximum measurement error of the scaling factor within 0.5%. The film images that are to be measured should be as large as possible so the effect of measurement error is decreased when the film values are scaled to life size.

Assuming that quality equipment (i.e., cameras, timing lights, film analyzer, and digitizer) and proper protocol have been used by the researcher, the accuracy of the displacement history (i.e., displacement plotted against time) of the digitized points in the photographic plane should be within 1% of the true value.

Other Considerations.   The *advantage* of the 2-D filming approach is its general simplicity of the filming procedure and subsequent analyses obtained. The *disadvantages* of a 2-D setup are that (a) it allows analyses only on a preselected single plane of movement and (b) the 2-D approach incorporates the dangers of perspective error for any nonplanar movements.

3-D CINEMATOGRAPHY

A number of acceptable 3-D filming methods are presently available to the researcher. A few of the more common 3-D approaches are those found in Martin and Pongratz (1974); Miller and Petak (1973); Shapiro (1978); Van Gheluwe (1978); and Woltring (1980). All of these techniques demand that their specific protocol be followed precisely.

Equipment Specifications.   A minimum of two motor-driven cameras but preferably more (three or four) equipped with a suitable mechanism for placing synchronized timing marks on the film in each camera should be used. If the cameras that are used do not provide for synchronized motor drive speed between both cameras, then one camera must be operated at a frame rate that is at least 50% in excess of the speed of the other camera. The camera with the slower filming rate will serve as the base line to which the frames of the higher speed camera can be matched. The matching is usually performed by filming a single timing device during the experiment.

If the particular 3-D protocol requires that the cameras be set up in a specific geometric configuration, then appropriate surveying methods and equipment should be used to make the alignment.

Calibration Procedures and Expected Reliability.   An accuracy check on the 3-D camera setup and synchronization system must be performed by the researcher for the particular study. This accuracy check can easily be performed by taking repeated length measurements on a rigid segment of known dimensions that moves in nonplanar fashion. The check also could be performed by flipping a wooden or metal rod into the air in the field of view of both cameras. The results of this accuracy evaluation test must be reported.

This will depend mostly on the care used in the experimental setup as well as on the quality of the equipment used. If the required protocol is followed, the investigator can expect the displacement history of a given point to be within 2% of the true value. The researcher will have an actual measure of the reliability of the employed 3-D filming system after conducting the test mentioned under Calibration Procedures.

Other Considerations.   The *advantage* of the 3-D filming approach is that perspective errors are minimized for any film measurements. Another advantage is that the 3-D analyses permit the measurement of a body's true movement in space. The *disadvantages* are (a) the extra setup procedures and additional filming equipment required and (b) the additional and more complex steps required in the analyses.

SINGLE-PLATE TECHNIQUES

As mentioned in chapter 2, the term single-plate technique is actually an umbrella term that includes (a) stroboscopy, (b) rotating-slit shutter, (c) light-streak photography, and (d) interrupted-light photography. The reader is referred to a paper by Smith (1975) for an excellent introductory discussion on single-plate techniques.

The protocol to be followed by these four techniques should be that which is used in any 2-D filming session. Some of the key points are

1. the filming plane in which the subject is to perform must be at right angles to the optical axis of the camera;
2. the key landmarks on the subject's body should be appropriately marked to provide a contrast to the background;
3. an object of known length should be filmed in the plane of motion at some time during the filming session; and
4. perspective error can be reduced by filming from as far away as possible, while at the same time employing a telephoto lens to maximize the size of the image.

For more specific testing protocol appropriate to the individual techniques, the following references are offered:

- For stroboscopy, the reader is referred to the paper by Merriman (1975).
- For the rotating-slit shutter technique, the reader is referred to the paper by Maier (1968).
- For light-streak pictures, the reader is referred to the paper by Hoecke and Gruendler (1975).
- For the interrupted-light technique, the reader is referred to the paper by Gutewort (1971).

Equipment Specifications.   The researcher should use a good quality lens and a camera (typically 35 mm) whose shutter can be set in the open position. If the stroboscopy technique is used, the strobe light should be a high quality research instrument that will allow the researcher to set the pulse width and the time interval between pulses.

Calibration Procedures and Expected Reliability.   As with all measurement techniques employed in research, the reliability of the data gathering system must be checked against a known value. This means the researcher must film a moving object whose displacement-time history is known. A disc rotating in the filming plane at a known constant angular velocity could provide the necessary data on which a reliability check on the measurement system could be performed. The displacement history (linear, angular) for planar movement of a measured point should be within 1% of the true value.

Other Considerations.   These systems are relatively inexpensive. By using polaroid film, rapid turn around time is available. However, the applications are quite limited for this type of data collection.

OPTOELECTRIC MOVEMENT MONITORING SYSTEM

A number of variations of these instruments are available today on the market and the researcher is advised to follow the procedure recommended by their respective designers closely.

Equipment Specifications.   Selspot is the trade name of one of the better known commercial models available. The reader is referred to the papers by Conati (1977), Gustafsson and Lanshammar (1977), and Woltring (1977) for a more thorough exposition of this particular model and second generation models. More recently, a less expensive system along the lines of Selspot has been developed by Wyss, Uozumi, and Polack (1981).

Another system on the market is the CODA-3 Movement Monitoring System. This system requires miniature prisms (< 2 g) instead of LEDs to be attached to the landmarks of interest. Further information on this system can be obtained from Movement Techniques Ltd., 17 South Street, Barrow-upon-Soar, Leicestershire, England, LE128LY. A Canadian system called Watsmart is being developed by Northern Digital in Waterloo, Ontario. This new monitoring system is a 3-D analysis package that will allow for the assessment of human motion. More information may be obtained by writing to Northern Digital, 415 Philip Street, Room 109, Waterloo, Ontario, N2L 3X2.

Calibration Procedures and Expected Reliability. As is true for all measurement systems employed by the researcher, the employed optoelectric system must be checked by the researcher for its reliability by comparing the system's output results with some known test criterion. The accuracy of this type of system should be within 1%, electronically speaking. However, the researcher should always treat with caution the output values that have been gained from an LED placed over soft tissue on a subject (e.g., as a hip joint marker).

At present, these types of systems lend themselves more to controlled laboratory conditions. The necessary equipment is usually quite sophisticated and expensive. Three-dimensional analysis can be performed, but additional equipment is necessary. This necessity leads to greater technical complexity as well as expense. As with other sophisticated equipment, a reasonably powerful computer is necessary for the data processing.

TELEVISION SYSTEMS

Although these systems have been in use for some time, currently much interest is in the development of this type of system because of the actual image that is available on the screen. This image provides the ability for subjective analysis, a benefit not inherent in the optoelectronic systems. Winter, Greenlaw, and Hobson (1972) provided an early system of television scanning for examining slow human motions such as gait. A newer system is provided by VICON (Computerized Kinematic Measurement System, Oxford Medilog, Inc., 11526 53rd St. N., Clearwater, FL, 33520) using reflective points for digitizing purposes. The technology in this area is progressing such that higher speed and resolution systems are quite feasible in the foreseeable future.

Calibration Procedures and Expected Reliability. The system should be checked for its accuracy by running a test on an object whose displacement history is known. The object could be a disc rotating at a known angular velocity. The accuracy of this system will be good as long as the

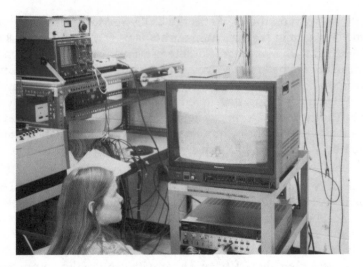

Figure 5.3 Use of TV system for walking analysis. Note reflective markers on monitor.

harmonic content of the signal remains relatively low. The content must remain low because the maximum sampling rate for most of the currently available television systems is 30 Hz. The Nyquist sampling theorem warns that the sampling rate must be at least twice the value of the highest frequency component contained in the pure signal. In practice, it is usually desirable to set the sampling rate in the order of 4 to 5 times the highest frequency component in order to get a satisfactory reproduction of the original signal. Thus a television system sampling at 30 Hz would not be suitable for measuring movement patterns above 8 to 10 Hz. The main use of the TV system is for walking analyses (Figure 5.3). Activities such as running and throwing have frequency components that are too high to be accurately analyzed with this system.

Sampling Rate and Data Smoothing

SAMPLING RATE

Lees (1980) suggested that the sampling rate need not exceed 50 Hz for most forms of voluntary human movement and may be lower for the majority of gross body activities. (The sampling rate is the number of frames analyzed per second, which can be considerably less than the actual filming rate. A high filming rate is often employed as a means of eliminating blurred film images. The cheaper alternative, of course, is to use a higher shutter factor). It has been a mistaken notion that measurement accuracy of any activity can be enhanced simply by increasing the number of frames analyzed per second (i.e., higher sampling rate). In truth, little, if any, additional information will be gained from sampling at a rate beyond 5 times the highest frequency component. This is not to say that a researcher is never justified in using sampling rates in excess of 50 Hz. For example, one could easily visualize experiments dealing with impact phenomena that would require a much greater sampling rate than 50 Hz. Keep in mind that the frequency domain of the expected data will dictate the sampling rate. The basic sampling theorem tells us that the sampling rate must be at least twice the frequency of the highest frequency component present in the pure signal (Hamming, 1977). This sampling rate is an absolute minimum theoretical value. In actual practice, choose a sampling rate 3 to 4 times the highest frequency component of interest.

DATA SMOOTHING

The computation of the velocity and acceleration history of an event by taking the first and second derivatives of the measured displacement data contains many dangers for the uninitiated. The higher frequency noise components, which result from imprecisions in human body parameter estimates and inaccuracies in the recording and digitizing processes, are greatly amplified when the higher order derivatives are computed on the displacement data. This amplification will lead to significant errors in the results unless the appropriate smoothing steps are taken. For a more detailed description of this particular error phenomenon, the reader is referred to Winter (1979a).

Currently, two accepted approaches are used to reduce or smooth out the errors that occur in the higher order derivatives. The first approach involves the use of a digital filter (e.g., Butterworth) followed by a finite difference technique (see Pezzack et al., 1977). The second approach involves the fitting of special mathematical functions to the displacement-time curves. An important property of these special mathematical functions is that they provide for easy computation of the higher order derivatives. At present only the Fourier series and spline functions have been shown to be acceptable for this second method of data smoothing in biomechanics. (See Hatze, 1981; Lees, 1980; Soudan & Dierskx, 1979; Wood & Jennings, 1979).

Direct Measurement Techniques

ACCELEROMETRY

The recommended protocol for a specific investigation will depend upon whether the investigator is measuring free motion in three dimensions or planar motion (one or two planes). One technique is outlined by Morris (1973); however, for greater accuracy and under certain circumstances the procedures of Padaonkar et al. (1975) are preferred. For constrained motion of mechanical analogues, (i.e., anthropometric dummies, head forms, or human body parts) the procedures outlined by Bishop (1976, 1977) or Norman et al. (1979) are recommended (See Figures 2.7 and 3.1).

Equipment Specifications. The following information should be considered when selecting appropriate accelerometers and for describing these devices in research reports:

- Type of accelerometer (strain gauge, piezoresistive, piezoelectric, etc.)
- Measuring range (m/s² or g)
- Frequency response (Hz)
- Resolution (m/s² or g)

Furthermore, reports must specify the number, arrangement, and fixation procedures that were employed, if applicable.

Calibration Procedures and Expected Reliability. In general, calibration is not necessary because most accelerometers are high precision instruments; however, calibration standards may be purchased from the manufacturer in most cases. A simple but crude calibration can be obtained by using gravitational acceleration as a standard (i.e., orient each axis vertically then horizontally to obtain 1 g or 9.8 m/s² output).

These devices are considered to be criterion measures of acceleration (e.g., Pezzack et al., 1977) but when poorly affixed (for instance, taped to skin) their output can be quite erroneous. Accelerometers should be mounted on rigid materials only and then attached securely to the desired body part or mounted within mechanical analogues. Accelerometers are not recommended for measuring whole body motions except for situations in which the purpose of a motion is to move in one direction such as bicycling, rowing, and wheeling (c.f. Cavagna, Saibene, & Margaria, 1963; Gage, 1964; Gersten et al., 1969; Winter, 1979b).

ELECTROGONIOMETRY AND POTENTIOMETRY

The recommended protocol for simple uniaxial electrogoniometers and potentiometers is outlined by Miller and Nelson (1973). Peat et al. (1976) have presented a modification that enables the measurement of angular displacement with respect to a gravity-based reference system. The procedures and principles of triaxial multijoint electrogoniometry are outlined by Chao (1978, 1980).

Equipment Specification.   Written reports concerning the use of potentiometers and electrogoniometers should include the following details:

- Orientation of axis (axes) and whether axis (axes) is coincident or
  external to joint axis (axes)
- Aligning procedures (i.e., self-aligning or not)
- Range of measurement (degrees or radians)
- Linearity (% full scale)
- Resolution (degrees or radians)
- Frequency response (Hz)

Calibration Procedures and Expected Reliability.   Linearity may be determined by comparing voltage output with the angle determined by a
manual goniometer or protractor. A more accurate and complex calibration
may be achieved using the methods described by Chao (1978, 1980).

These devices are typically custom-made and therefore reliability and accuracy are dependent upon the design considerations made by the investi-
gator(s). These devices are, however, generally considered to be criterion
measures of joint angular displacements. Chao (1980) discusses the accuracy that special design-calibrated electrogoniometers can achieve. Note
that when angular velocities and accelerations are required, analogue or
digital techniques may be employed to obtain these measurements.

Other considerations.   Electrogoniometers and potentiometers are used
primarily to study the relative or absolute motion of one or a few joints.
They are not recommended for detailed kinematic studies of complex
human motion because they do not measure with respect to an inertial
(Newtonian) frame of reference. Further data such as photographs or cine-
films are required to enable the quantification of complex human motions
for most kinematic analyses.

Physical Properties of the Limbs and the Total Body

The approximation of the segmental physical properties must be regarded with respect to the type of application for which they are intended.
Most of the methods used in living subjects require sophisticated equipment or involve lengthy procedures; much time is usually required from
the subject. Because these methods have not been fully validated and are
still very restricted in their applicability for some of the body segments,
whether these approaches should be recommended to the investigators
whose first purpose consists in evaluating human performance from cinematographic analysis is doubtful.

In this case, it appears preferable to recommend the norms or regression equations obtained from cadavers. Furthermore, it is not known if such approximations are really less valid than the approximations obtained from the mentioned techniques that are applied to living subjects. The norms developed by Dempster (1955) for segmental weights and centers of gravity and the norms established by Plagenhoef (1971) which are based on Dempster's data for radius of gyration would be recommended because they constitute the only source available from cadaver data where all properties are derived. Only parts of this information are available in other studies.

A synthesis of this information found in Williams and Lissner and revised by LeVeau (1977) includes

1. the surface landmarks associated with joint centers (p. 208);
2. the segmental weight/body weight ratios (p. 211);
3. the center of mass/segment length ratios to the proximal end (p. 212);
4. the radius of gyration as a percentage of segment length for both the proximal and distal ends (p. 213).

Expected Validity.   The validity of this information remains to be established. Validity is yet to be established for all the existing techniques applied to cadavers and/or living subjects. The problem is related to the assumptions required.

Muscular Forces and Moments and Joint Reaction Forces

These types of measurement imply a modeling approach and the use of cinematographical techniques. The model is simplified when only the net muscular moments are obtained. In this case, the free body diagram of the forces involved in the modeled segment excludes the muscular forces; these forces are resolved into a joint reaction force and a resultant couple. The problems then can be solved by applying dynamic equations. The reader is referred to Winter (1979a) for a description of this type of model applied to planar motions. For determining if the resultant moment is eccentric or concentric, the angular velocity of the limbs must be evaluated. This approach is presented by Robertson and Winter (1980). The following information must be provided as input data: (a) the inertial parameters; mass, center of mass, moment of intertia, and joint center, (b) the kinematics of motion; absolute linear and angular accelerations, and (c) in some cases, ground reaction forces and their location relative to the joint center.

In the measures of muscular forces and joint reaction forces, the model is further complicated by the fact that all muscles must be identified with their direction of pull and their sites of attachment relative to the joint center. To remove the indeterminations and solve the problem, optimization techniques are used. The simplest one appears to be linear programming (Dantzig, 1968). Each type of problem is specific in nature with regard to the boundary values or constraints, the hypothesis on muscle actions, and the optimization characteristics.

Refer to Schultz and Andersson (1981) for a comprehensive description of the modeling approaches with applications to measurements of loads on the lumbar spine and the contraction forces in the trunk muscles likely to be encountered in different physical activities.

The following pieces of equipment may be required for this type of analysis:

1. Force platforms (see this chapter, Force Platforms and Pressure Platforms).
2. Cinematography techniques applied to planar or tridimensional motions including smoothing and numerical differentiation procedures (see this chapter, Imaging Technique and Smoothing and Differentiation Technique).

Calibration Procedures and Expected Reliability.   The calibration procedures are those associated with the techniques mentioned in the preceding section. The validity of muscular forces and moments and joint reaction forces obtained by the prescribed models has not been fully demonstrated. One can only speak about partial validity examined by means of electromyography (for forces), of internal pressure measurements (for joint reaction forces), and the consistency of the motion patterns with muscular motions. The problem of validation is well recognized by researchers. Schultz and Andersson (1981) mentioned that the range of loads experienced by the body is so large that in spite of the uncertainties introduced in the models, these models can provide solutions for practical problems. However, investigating the relative effects of the recognized sources of error on the changes in the dynamics of motion would be interesting. For instance, what happens if the segmental mass and moment of inertia are underestimated or overestimated by 5%? These effects could be examined in a systematic manner and they could give information about the validity of some basic assumptions.

Force and Pressure Transducers

In this section, the following topics will be presented: (a) transducers, (b) force platforms, and (c) pressure platforms.

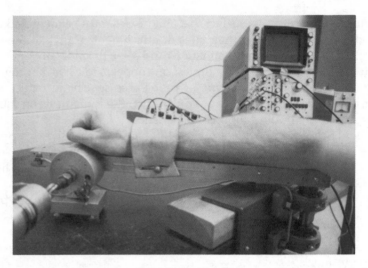

Figure 5.4   Force transducers-(LVDT) used to measure elbow flexion and extension isometric strength (muscle movement).

TRANSDUCERS

In order to measure the force exerted by the body on its external environment or some other mechanical parameter, transducers are required. A transducer is a device that provides a suitable output in response to a specific measurand (Figure 5.4). A large number of transducers exist that are classified according to the transduction elements: capacitative, electromagnetic, inductive, photoconductive, photovoltaic, piezoelectric, resistive (e.g., strain gauges), and so on. The force platform includes an assembly incorporating some transduction elements, usually of piezoelectric or strain gauge types. Very recently, advances have been made in the design of pressure platforms with capacitative or peizoelectric transduction elements. The general characteristics of transducers and the general criteria for their selection are discussed in this section.

Equipment Specifications (Characteristics of Transducers).   The static and dynamic performance characteristics of transducers are very important to understand when applying any transducer for a specific function. The information contained herein was taken in part from the *Handbook of Transducers for Electronic Measuring Systems* (1969).

Calibration Procedures and Expected Reliability of Static Performance Characteristics.   The transducer characteristics are determined during calibration at room conditions (temperature of 25 ± 10 °C, humidity of 90% or less and ambient relative pressure of 88.0 to 108.4 KPa). The calibration test consists of applying to the transducer some known values of a measurand and of recording the corresponding output value. When this is done once in an ascending mode and once in a descending mode, a calibration cycle is performed.

Hysteresis. The maximum difference in any pair of output readings (one in the ascending mode and one in the descending mode) during one cycle of calibration is referred to as the hysteresis of the transducer and is expressed as percentage of full-scale output.

Linearity. A transducer is considered linear when the calibration data approach a specified straight line. Several definitions for the specified straight line can be found but the most commonly used is the line obtained by joining the end points of the calibration curve. In this case, one refers to end-point linearity. Linearity is expressed in plus or minus a percentage of full-scale output.

Transverse Sensitivity. This is the response of a transducer to measurand values applied in axes transverse to the sensing axis. The transverse sensitivity should be null in theory.

Repeatability. This is the ability of the transducer to reproduce output readings during two or more successive cycles of calibration. Repeatability is expressed as the maximum difference between output readings at any measurand value and is expressed in percentage of full-scale output.

Dynamic Performance Characteristics. When a measurand is used in conditions where rapid measurand variations occur, the dynamic characteristics of the transducer must be established. In dynamic calibration, the measurand is made to vary in some specific manner (sine wave, square wave, etc.), and the output is recorded as a function of time.

Frequency Response. When the measurand is applied to the transducer as a sine wave over a given frequency range, the output/measurand amplitude ratio may change with frequency. This provides information with respect to frequency response. Frequency response is expressed as "within $\pm x$ percent from y to z Hz" and is referred to a specific reference frequency within the range and to a specific amplitude level of reference.

Response Time. When a step change of the measurand is applied to the transducer, the time required for the corresponding output change to reach 63% of its final value is the time constant of the transducer. The response time is the time required to reach high percentages (for instance, 90%, 98%, or 99%) of this final value.

Damping. The upper limit of frequency response and the response-time characteristics are affected by the energy dissipation properties of the transducer. An underdamped transducer will produce an overshoot in the output value and some oscillations will be observed about the final value. On the other hand, an overdamped transducer will produce a time lag before the final value will be reached.

Vibrations.   As vibrations in a specified range of frequencies and amplitudes are applied to a transducer, amplified vibration components (resonances) can occur within narrow frequency ranges. The vibration error is the maximum change in output when vibration levels with determined frequencies and amplitudes are applied to the transducer.

Other Considerations.   The selection of a transducer usually involves the following basic considerations:

1. What is the real purpose of the measurement?
2. What range of the measurand is expected in the applications?
3. What is the accuracy required in the measurements?
4. What are the lower and upper limits of frequency response or response time needed in the data?
5. What are the environmental conditions in which the transducer will be used?
6. What transduction principle should be utilized?
7. Is the cost of the transducer compatible with the necessity for the measurement?
8. What is the weight of the transducer?

FORCE PLATFORMS

A force platform is a device designed to measure the forces exerted by a body on an external surface, namely the force platform.

Design.   The force platform includes the transducers, the amplifiers, and the recording equipment. The most common types of transducers in force platforms are strain gauges and piezoelectric quartzes. The transducer converts the mechanical entity (force) into another measurable form (electrical). The amplifier is a device that increases the magnitude of the signal to facilitate data recording and processing. The display is the mode of representation of the signal (chart recorder, oscilloscope, magnetic tape, etc.).

Basic Considerations in Design and Utilization.   The platform must be designed to accommodate foot contact with a minimum necessity of targeting the platform (Figure 5.5). The force platform should possess the following characteristics to provide valid measures of force: adequate sensitivity, high linearity, low hysteresis, and low cross-talk between the different axes. Special care must be taken to eliminate the interference associated with cable aberrations, electrical conductance, and temperature and humidity variations. The amplifier must be stable, linear, and pro-

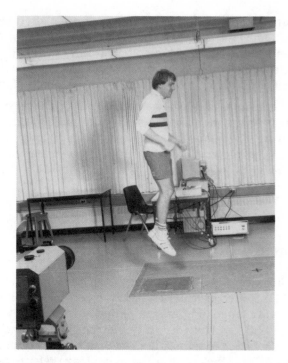

Figure 5.5 Ground reaction force analysis of vertical jump using an "AMTI" force platform.

vide adequate gain. Moreover, choosing an appropriate recording system is important; for instance, it is of no use to match a transducer of high frequency response to a recorder with low frequency response.

The structure of the platform must be relatively light and designed in a way to provide high stiffness and a sufficiently high natural frequency. From the theory of elasticity, the platform may be represented by a simple model such as a simply supported beam with the load at the center and the natural frequency evaluated from the known equations:

$$\delta = \frac{P\ell^3}{48EI} \; ; \; K = \frac{P}{\delta} \; ; \; f = \frac{1}{2\pi} \sqrt{\frac{K}{M}}$$

Where δ = deflection, P = load, ℓ = length of the beam between supports (m), E = modulus of elasticity of the beam material (N/m²), I = second moment of area of the cross-section of the beam (m⁴), K = stiffness of the system, f = natural frequency (Hz), and M = mass of frame plus force platform (kg).

This analysis has been presented by Seedhom (1980) in relation to the design of force platforms.

One important consideration in locating the force platform is the vibrations transmitted by traffic or machinery. These vibrations may substantially contaminate the signal. Therefore, it is recommended that the researcher locate the platform on the ground floor and mount it in a concrete block so that it will be totally isolated from the foundations of the building.

Calibration Procedures and Expected Reliability. The preceding information on transducers and force platforms may guide those people interested in having the platform designed for their own needs. This information is also relevant for the potential buyer of manufactured platforms. Several types of force platforms were presented in the section on kinetics (chapter 3) under Testing Procedures for Ground Reaction Forces and Pressure Distribution. The Kistler platform has been extensively used in research and provides valid and reliable data for the analysis of dynamic situations in sport. The Kistler platform is based on piezoelectric transduction by means of quartz discs. The platform provides a very high range of force measurements (Fx and Fy: -10 to 10 kN; Fz: -10 to 20 kN), low threshold, high sensitivity, high linearity ($< \pm 0.5\%$ FSO), low hysteresis ($< 0.5\%$ of FSO), low cross-talk (less than 2%), very high natural frequency (> 1k Hz), a wide range of operating temperature (from -20 to 70 °C), and low weight (41 kg). However, piezoelectric platforms may not be the most appropriate ones to use for the evaluation of forces in quasi-static motions, and if this is the case the researcher may prefer to buy a strain-gauged platform.

PRESSURE PLATFORMS

A pressure platform is a device designed to measure the pressure distribution beneath the foot. Presently, no commercial pressure platforms are designed for sport applications. All the information in the literature pertaining to pressure distribution measures was obtained from different types of platforms designed for use in the specific research laboratories where this type of research was conducted.

A successful approach to pressure platform design is one provided by Hennig et al. (1980). The platform is based on piezoelectric transduction with ceramic materials; the ceramic materials are made piezoelectric by polarization in a high electric field at temperatures near the Curie point (piezoceramics). Refer to Hennig et al. (1980) for a complete description of the design.

Calibration Procedures and Expected Reliability. The performance characteristics of the platform are excellent: high linearity ($< 2\%$), low hysteresis ($< 1\%$), a wide range of measures (1500 kPa for each transducer element covering an area of 4 mm $\times$ 4 mm) a high response frequency (> 2 kHz for each transducer), and high resolution (< .05 kPa). The pressure distribution can be recorded in discrete form and the tridimensional display can be provided. Cavanagh and Michiyoshi (1980) described this display of data in a more complete form. The pressure estimate for each transducer was plotted as the component normal to the plane of a shoe outline in such a way that a continuous surface was formed where the height of the surface was proportional to pressure.

Impulses and Momenta

LINEAR IMPULSES

Linear impulses exerted by the athlete on the ground and the subsequent *momenta* resulting from impulses can be evaluated at any moment during motion by means of force-time measurements and integration procedures. The force-time records are provided by a force platform. If the initial velocity is known, the curve of velocity development as a function of time may be calculated. The evaluation of the initial velocity is the problem of major concern. For motions initiated from rest, the intial velocity is assumed null; otherwise, the initial velocity must be approximated (a) by two photoelectric cells a very small distance apart and positioned very near the force platform at the hip height and (b) by numerical differentiation of the displacement-time data of the body's center of gravity.

ANGULAR IMPULSES

Angular impulses exerted on the ground are evaluated with force-time measurements and the measures of the lever arms of forces with respect to the body's center of gravity. In that case, cinematography, force platform techniques, and integration procedures must be used in combination. The subsequent change in *angular momentum* is evaluated from the angular impulse curve. If the initial angular momentum ($I\omega$) is null, then the angular velocity is assumed to be null, and it is easy to measure the angular momentum at any moment during the angular impulse; otherwise, both the values of the moment of inertia and angular velocity must be approximated at the initiation of impulse. The procedures developed by Ramey and Yang (1981) are recommended in this case.

AIRBORNE ACTIVITIES

For airborne types of activities, the linear momentum may be measured by evaluating the linear momentum at the end of the takeoff phase from the integration of force-time records with the force platform. Then the initial velocities at takeoff may be evaluated, and the equations of kinematics for parabolic flight are used to predict certain parameters such as the vertical rise of the center of gravity.

The angular momentum is constant during airborne activities. The procedures developed by Ramey and Yang (1981) seem the most appropriate ones. They used a model that can be extended to any number of body segments and that can be applied to tridimensional analyses of motion.

Equipment Specifications. The following pieces of equipment may be required for this type of analysis:

- Force platforms (see this chapter, Force and Pressure Transducers).
- Cinematography techniques applied to planar or tridimensional motions and smoothing and differentiation procedures (see this chapter under the headings Imaging Technique, and Smoothing and Differentiation Techniques).
- Integrators incorporated into the platform assembly or numerical integration procedures. The most commonly used are Simpson's rule and the trapezoidal rule. These numerical integration procedures may be very precise to integrate the force-time data but the use of a high sampling rate is recommended; 50 Hz is usually appropriate.

Calibration Procedures and Expected Reliability. The calibration procedures are those associated with the techniques mentioned in Equipment Specifications. The validity of the linear impulse and momentum may be established by comparing the kinematic parameters (maximum rise in center of gravity, time of flight, and horizontal distance) during the flight phase predicted from the takeoff velocities obtained from the impulse curves to the kinematic parameters actually measured by cinematography. These measures are usually highly valid if the force platform presents high performance characteristics; moreover, the numerical integration procedures are usually highly valid. The validity of the angular momentum determined from segmental modeling has not yet been fully established. Several assumptions are imposed on these models whose validity is still questionable: for instance, the physical properties of the segments.

BODY SEGMENT AND TOTAL BODY ENERGIES AND MECHANICAL WORK OUTPUT

Note that mechanical efficiency is easily calculated from equation 3-24 (see page 48) if the total mechanical work output and metabolic cost are known. Metabolic measurement techniques can be found in many articles, one of them, "Physiological Testing of the Elite Athlete," is a Canadian Association of Sport Sciences publication (MacDougall, Wenger, & Green, 1982). For more detail on the mechanical work output and body segment energy calculations and interpretations, refer to Pierrynowski, Norman, and Winter (1981). A discussion of issues concerning the concept of mechanical efficiency is found in articles by Winter (1979b) and more recently by Williams and Cavanagh (1983).

The instantaneous energy level of each body segment can be calculated, for example, in a model of a skier (Figure 5.6). From this, one can construct the mechanical energy time history during one movement cycle, in this case, from pushoff of the left foot to pushoff of the right foot or some other convenient step identifier. Equations 5-1 and 5-2 define the mathematical process

$$TE_{ij} = M_i gh_{ij} + \frac{1}{2} M_i v^2{}_{Gij} + \frac{1}{2} I_{Gi} w^2{}_{ij} \qquad (5\text{-}1)$$

$$TE_{ij} = PE_{ij} + TKE_{ij} + RKE_{ij} \qquad (5\text{-}2)$$

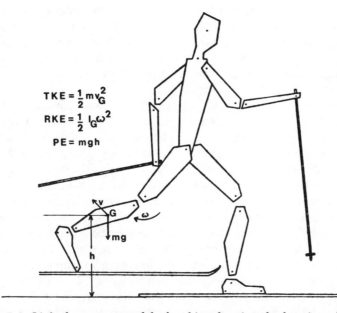

Figure 5.6 Linked segment model of a skier showing the location of the center of gravity (G) of the swinging lower leg, its transitional velocity (v), its rotational velocity (ω), its height above the ground (h), its mass (m), the gravitational constant (g) and the related energy components, Translational Kinetic Energy (TKE), Rotational Kinetic Energy (RKE), and Potential Energy, (PE).

where i, j = segment, time; TE = Total energy; PE = potential energy above some datum (i.e., the ground); TKE = translatory kinetic energy; RKE = rotational kinetic energy; M = segment mass; g = gravitational constant; h = vertical position above an arbitrary datum; v = translatory velocity of center of gravity; I = moment of inertia about center of gravity; ω = angular velocity.

Equations 5-1 and 5-2 indicate that component energy curves (PE, TKE, and RKE) can be constructed for each body segment, and a total energy curve for that segment can be constructed by adding the component curves. In Figure 5.7, the curves labelled RE_1, PE_1, and KE_1 are the component energy curves for one step cycle for segment 1, the right leg; those with the subscript 2 are for the trunk. The changes in energy level of each of these component curves can be thought of as the work done on that segment to produce changes in rotational velocity, in translational velocity, and in vertical displacement, reflected in ΔRE, ΔKE, and ΔPE, respectively.

Adding these component energy changes separately in this way, segment by segment, produces a total work output value, which implicitly assumes no transfers between potential and kinetic energy or transfers of energy from body segment to segment. This assumption is unrealistic physiologically and biomechanically. The calculation is useful, however, as a baseline value against which the extent of exploitation of low metabolic cost energy transfers by an athlete can be ascertained. This work output calculation is labelled W_N in Figure 5.7.

As inferred above, energy can be transferred between kinetic and potential forms in the manner of a pendulum. These transfers are accounted for if the three component energy curves are first added to produce a single total energy curve for that segment. These total energy curves for the right leg and trunk are labelled TE_1 and TE_2, respectively. The work done on the segment can be calculated from the sum of the absolute changes in the total segment energy curves. The implicit assumption is that energy transfers within body segments are possible, but dealing with each segment independently of the others implies no transfers between segments. The work done by all of the segments is then calculated as W_W in Figure 5.7.

Finally, a total body energy curve (TE_B in Figure 5.7) can be constructed by adding the total energy curves for each segment (TE_1 + TE_2, etc.). This curve finishes at an energy level higher than that at which it began primarily because of the slight elevation in terrain over the step cycle, shown in the example curves (about 0.2 m), giving rise to a net increase in potential energy.

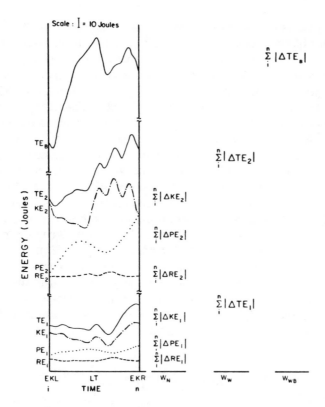

Figure 5.7 Body segment, segment component, and total body energy curves, and corresponding work terms for cross-country skier. Average velocity of step 5.24 m/s.

EKL, (EKR)	— end of kick of left (right) leg; leg starts downward
LT	— legs together
RE, PE, KE, TE	— rotational kinetic, potential, translational kinetic and total energy
TE_B	— total body energy
TE_1 and TE_2	— total segment energy, right leg and trunk, respectively
W_N, W_W, W_{WB}	— total work output assuming (a) No energy transfers, (b) transfers Within, (c) transfers Within and Between segments, respectively

See text for further explanation of terms. Note that in this figure the rotational kinetic energy (RKE) is labelled (RE), the translational kinetic energy (TKE) is labelled (KE), and the total segment or body energies are labelled (TE).

Rising phases of energy level in the curve TE (and the other curves) represent phases of positive work. Falling energy levels indicate phases of negative work. Both positive and negative work cost metabolic energy although positive work appears to be about 3 to 5 times more costly than negative work (Abbott, Bigland, & Ritchie, 1952; Margaria, 1968). The total work done is equal to the sum of the absolute energy changes in curve TE_B and is labelled W_{WB} in Figure 5.7. The implicit assumption (and reality) is that energy transfers within body segments and between adjacent segments occur in human movement. To accommodate the metabolic cost of negative work, adding both the rises and the falls in energy level is necessary (c.f. Winter, 1979b). Some authors (e.g., Cavagna, Saibene, & Margaria, 1964; Ralston & Lukin, 1969) included only the phases of positive work in their estimates of work output. Yet others have proposed constraints on the extent to which transfers of energy between segments are biomechanically feasible (c.f. Williams & Cavanagh, 1983). No definitive statement as to the most appropriate calculation can be made at present.

No unequivocal position can be taken at present and in the face of a degree of uncertainty we propose that W_{WB} is the mechanical work output value for the total body that most reasonably represents physiological conditions. Equation 5-3 is the numerical expression for this calculation

$$W_{WB} = \sum_{j=1}^{n} \left| \sum_{i=1}^{s} (\Delta TE_{ij}) \right| = \sum_{i=1}^{n} |\Delta TE_B| \qquad (5\text{-}3)$$

where W_{WB} = work done assuming energy transfers within and between segments, n = film frames (time), and TE_B = total body energy.

Equipment Specifications.

1. Kinematic input for the equations can be obtained from film, light emitting diodes (e.g., Selspot), or any other source that yields body segment displacement and velocity information in an absolute reference frame. See the section on imaging techniques.
2. Appropriate smoothing and differentiation techniques must be applied to the data. See the section on smoothing and differentiation techniques.
3. Body segment masses, mass moments of inertia, locations of segment, and total body centers of gravity and joint centers are obtained according to the methods proposed in the section on body segment parameters.
4. A camera, good film digitizing system, a computer with an adequate core for the model selected, and a well debugged software package written to accommodate the equations for the analysis are required.

5. The calibration procedures are those associated with the techniques mentioned in Actual Protocol for calculating mechanical efficiency.
6. The accuracy and reliability of the mechanical energy and work output values depend on the quality of the input kinematic and body segment parameter data. Errors in the linear velocities of the segments are particularly serious. The filter cutoff frequencies chosen, if the data are smoothed in this way, can affect the size of the work output appreciably because small phase shifts in the individual curves have a substantial effect on the sum of the curves even when the shapes and amplitudes of the component curves appear similar.

Error increases if the film is of poor quality, the images are small, or the location of some joint markers has to be estimated because they are hidden from the view of the camera for substantial portions of the movement cycle.

Reasonably stable data are obtained from well learned movement patterns such as walking by averaging at least two complete strides (e.g., two cycles from right heel contact to right heel contact). An average of three strides (movement cycles) is better, but averaging four does not seem to produce an appreciably different mean than averaging three (Grainger, Norman, Winter, & Bobet, 1983).

Other Considerations.

1. The equations presented are for two-dimensional motion. Three-dimensional analyses of this nature are not yet routinely done in most biomechanics laboratories. In principle, however, the approach could be applied in three dimensions.
2. **CAUTION:** The implicit assumptions about energy transfers within and between body segments that appear in the data depend entirely on how the matrix of the energies of the various body segments and the energy components (PE, TKE, RKE) are added across the time of the movement cycle. It is *essential* that the additions in the computer program are done according to the equations presented or an equivalent.

INTERSEGMENTAL POWER ANALYSIS

The methods for determining the various rates of energy inflow and outflow to the body segments are described by Elftman (1939), Quanbury, Winter, & Reimer (1975), and Robertson and Winter (1980). A graphical method of illustrating the results of this type of analysis, applied to walking, is presented by Winter and Robertson (1978).

Equipment Specifications.   The computations for performing this type of analysis require (a) kinematics of the joints and net forces and moments of force at the joints (see this chapter, Muscular Forces and Moments and Joint Reaction Forces) and (b) segment total energies (see chapter 3, Mechanical Energy, Work, and Efficiency). This analysis is based upon numerical computations and so requires no specific equipment except those associated with obtaining the above mentioned measures.

Calibration Procedures. A method of validating the computations performed by this analysis should be undertaken to assess the magnitude and occurrence of errors. A method for achieving this objective is described and illustrated by Robertson and Winter (1980) for walking analyses. Cappozzo, Figura, and Marchetti (1976) describe another less specific form of this validation that compares the total work done by the muscle moments of force with the changes in total mechanical energy of the body.

Reliability of this type of analysis applied to sporting activities is still to be determined because, to date, the analysis has been restricted to the study of walking. For walking studies, the accuracy was found to be quite high for free swinging segments, but significant errors were introduced during transient events such as footstrike and toeoff. Errors during free swinging motions were less than 5% of peak power (Robertson & Winter, 1980) but were considerably higher for the foot segment during contact with the ground. The shank and thigh segments showed errors as high as 20% of peak power during periods of ground contact.

Neuromuscular Measurement (EMG)

The first step in neuromuscular testing involves locating the motor point: for example, the point where the main trunk nerve enters the muscle (Cohen & Brunlik, 1976) to be studied. The purpose of motor point assessment is to identify the best site for electrode placement. A square wave stimulator, delivering pulses of 300 ms duration at intervals of 500 ms is used to determine motor points. Once the subject has been properly positioned, the dispersive electrode is wet and placed in contact with the skin of the same extremity as the one tested to prevent electrical current from being conducted to other parts of the body. To lessen skin resistance during motor point localization, the skin and the exploring electrode are kept wet throughout this procedure. The exploring electrode is applied as close as possible to the hypothetical motor point of the muscle (Walthard & Tchicaloff, 1971) (Figure 5.8). Without removing the testing electrode from the skin, the electrical stimulator is set to the "on" position and the intensity of stimulation is gradually increased until a muscle contraction is observed. Once a contraction is observed, the voltage is reduced until contraction is barely visible. With this reduced current, the testing electrode explores adjacent skin areas until the greatest muscular contraction with a mini-

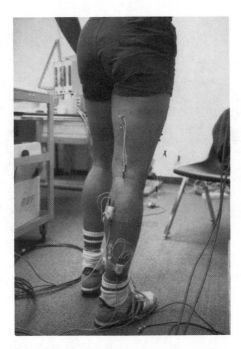

Figure 5.8 Example of EMG electrodes on leg muscle.

mum amount of voltage is observed. The motor point is then the location on the muscle where the smallest amount of voltage causes the greatest contraction. The location of the motor point is marked.

The next step in neuromuscular testing involves preparing the skin to lower its resistance before applying the electrodes. The resistance of the unprepared skin varies over a wide range, depending on skin site, subject, time and skin preparation (see International Society of Electrophysiological Kinesiology [ISEK] guidelines, Appendix C). In order to minimize the influence of this complex resistance on the signal, ISEK (Appendix C) recommends using high input resistance amplifiers. In the case when this type of equipment is not available, skin preparation is recommended to lower its resistance (Walthard & Tchicaloff, 1971). The electrodes are then ready to be put in place using collars and electrode paste (see Appendix C). The pickup electrode should be placed directly over the motor point, and the reference electrode should be placed a few centimeters distally from the pickup electrode. For amplifier and recorder selection, see ISEK guidelines (Appendix C). As far as EMG quantification is concerned, all neuromuscular parameters suggested can be derived from the raw electromyographical signals which require no quantification of the signal (Figure 5.9).

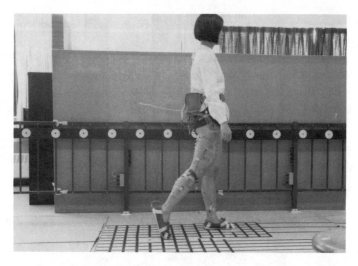

Figure 5.9   Sixteen channel EMG telemetry of leg muscle activity during walking, integrated with force measurement from two force plates (squared area on floor).

Summary

Many techniques, problems, and limitations have been discussed in this chapter. Again, the list and the descriptions are not exhaustive, but they represent an overview of many of the testing protocols available today. In choosing the correct approach to testing an athlete or group of athletes many considerations must be taken into account. The multidisciplinary approach provides many advantages in terms of breadth of understanding. An essential part of any investigative team is a qualified biomechanist who understands the type of testing to be performed, and who also has at his or her disposal the instrumentation and computer software necessary to perform the testing.

A consideration that must be seriously addressed is the funding of a testing or research project. By way of a guideline to this problem a sample budget is provided in Appendix D for a simple filming project. The costs are, if anything, conservative. Because of the sophistication in equipment and personnel necessary for good, sound information to be generated, the price is rising steadily. It is hoped that the protocols described in this chapter will be followed and that the budget will not be the major consideration in undertaking a research or testing project. Good work is expensive, but it is also money well spent, not wasted.

Appendix A

International System of Units (SI)*

*Canadian Standards Association-Toronto, 1973

International System of Units (SI)—Canadian Standards Association Outline

	Quantity	Abbreviation	Unit	Symbol	Expression
Base units	length	ℓ	meter	m	
	mass	M	kilogram	kg	
	time	t	second	s	
	electric current		ampere	A	
Supplementary units	plane angle		radian	rad	
	solid angle		steradian	sr	
Derived units having special names	frequency		hertz	Hz	s^{-1}
	force	F	newton	N	$kg \cdot m/s^2$
	pressure, stress		pascal	Pa	N/m^2
	work	U			
	energy	E			
	quantity of heat		joule	J	$N \cdot m$
	power	P	watt	W	J/s
	electric charge		coulomb	C	$A \cdot s$
	electromotive force		volt	V	W/A
	electric resistance		ohm	Ω	V/A
	electric capacitance		farad	F	C/V
	magnetic flux		weber	Wb	$V \cdot s$
	inductance		henry	H	Wb/A

	Quantity	Symbol	Unit name	Unit symbol	Value
Other derived units	area		square meter		m²
	volume		cubic meter		m³
	velocity-angular	ω	radian per second		rad/s
	velocity-linear	ν	meter per second		m/s
	acceleration-angular	α	radian per second squared		rad/s²
	acceleration-linear	a	meter per second squared		m/s²
	density (mass per unit volume)		kilogram per cubic meter		kg/m³
	moment of force	τ	newton meter		N · m
	displacement-linear	d	meter		m
	displacement-angular	θ	radian		rad
Special names	time		minute	min	60 s
			hour	h	3600 s
			day	d	86,400 s
	plane angle		degree	°	$(\pi/180)$ rad
			minute	'	$(\pi/10{,}800)$ rad
			second	''	$(\pi/648{,}000)$ rad
	volume		liter	1	1 dm³
	temperature		degree Celcius	°C	273.15 K
	mass		tonne	t	1000 kg
	momentum-linear	H			kg · m/s
	momentum-angular	h			kg · m²/s
	moment of inertia	I			kg · m²
	impulse-linear	J			N · s
	impulse-angular				N · m · s

Multiplying factor	Prefix	Symbol
$1,000,000,000,000 = 10^{12}$	tera	T
$1,000,000,000 = 10^{9}$	giga	G
$1,000,000 = 10^{6}$	mega	M
$1,000 = 10^{3}$	kilo	k
$100 = 10^{2}$	hecto	h
$10 = 10^{1}$	deca	da
$0.1 = 10^{-1}$	deci	d
$0.01 = 10^{-2}$	centi	c
$0.001 = 10^{-3}$	milli	m
$0.000,001 = 10^{-6}$	micro	π
$0.000,000,001 = 10^{-9}$	nano	n
$0.000,000,000,001 = 10^{-12}$	pico	p

Appendix B

Policy Statement Regarding the Use of Human Subjects and Informed Consent*

By law, any experimental subject or clinical patient who is exposed to possible physical, psychological, or social injury must give informed consent prior to participating in a proposed project. Informed consent can be defined as the knowing consent of an individual or his legally authorized representative so situated as to be able to exercise free power of choice without undue inducement or any element of force, fraud, deceit, duress, or other form of constraint or coercion.

The Editorial Board of *Medicine and Science in Sports* requires that all appropriate steps be taken in obtaining the informed consent of any and all human subjects employed by investigators submitting manuscripts for review and possible publication. In most cases, informed consent should be obtained by having the subject read a document (an Informed Consent Form) presenting all information pertinent to the investigation or project and affixing a signature indicating that the document has been read and consent given to participation under the conditions described therein. The document should be so written as to be easily understandable to the subjects and provided in a language in which the subject is fluent.

Investigators are requested to consider the following items for inclusion in an Informed Consent Form as appropriate to the particular project:

1. A general statement of the background of the project and the project objectives.
2. A fair explanation of the procedures to be followed and their purposes, identification of any procedures which are experimental, and description of any and all risks attendant to the procedures.

---

*Reprinted with permission of the American College of Sports Medicine and Medicine and Science in Sports.

3. A description of any benefits reasonably to be expected and, in the case of treatment, disclosure of any appropriate alternative procedures that might be advantageous for the subject.
4. An offer to answer any queries of the subject concerning procedures or other aspects of the project.
5. An instruction that the subject is free to withdraw consent and to discontinue participation in the project or activity at any time without prejudice to the subject.
6. An instruction that, in the case of questionnaires and interviews, the subject is free to deny answer to specific items or questions.
7. An instruction that, if services or treatment are involved in the setting or context of the project, neither will they be enhanced nor diminished as a result of the subject's decision to volunteer or not to volunteer participation in the project.
8. An explanation of the procedures to be taken to insure the confidentiality of the data and information to be derived from the subject. If subjects are to be identified by name in the manuscript, permission for same should be included in the Informed Consent Form or obtained in writing at a later date.

If the subject is to be videotaped or photographed in any manner, this must be disclosed in the Informed Consent Form. The subject must be advised as to who will have custody of such videotapes or photographs, who will have access to the tapes or photographs, how the tapes or photographs are to be used, and what will be done with them when the study is completed.

The informed consent document must not contain any exculpatory language or any other waiver of legal rights releasing, or appearing to release, an investigator, project director, or institution from liability. At the bottom of the form, provision should be made for the signature of the subject (and date signed) and/or a legally authorized representative. It is generally advisable to precede this with a statement to the effect that the subject and/or representative have read the statement and do understand. In the case of minors, one or both parents should sign as appropriate. For minors of sufficient maturity, signatures should be obtained from the subject and the parent(s).

The Editorial Board endorses the Declaration of Helsinki of the World Medical Association as regards the conduct of clinical research. Physicians are expected to comply with the principles set forth in this declaration when research involves the use of patients. In the case of psychological research, investigators will be expected to comply with the principles established by the American Psychological Association. These principles are presented in the publication, "Ethical Principles in the Conduct of Research with Human Subjects" (American Psychological Association, Washington, DC, 1973).

It will not be necessary for an author to describe in the manuscript the specific steps that were taken to obtain informed consent, to insure confidentiality of results, or to protect the privacy rights of participating subjects. It will be satisfactory for the author to indicate by a phrase that, "Informed consent was obtained from the subjects," or similar. It will be understood by the editors that such a statement indicates the author's guarantee of compliance with the directives presented above.

Appendix C

Units, Terms and Standards in the Reporting of EMG Research*

Authors' Note

This report is the final report of an ISEK Ad Hoc Committee that was formed in 1977 to deal with the problems arising from inconsistent and erroneous terms and units in the reporting of EMG research. The Committee has addressed this problem at all levels, from the electrophysiological terminology right through to the more common processing techniques. Also, the Committee makes some recommendations regarding technical standards that should be aimed for by all researchers. This report has evolved from the First Interim Report presented at the 4th Congress of ISEK in Boston in August 1979, from meetings held with researchers at the Congress, and from many personal discussions held over the past few years. The document presents not only the fundamental theoretical and physiological relationships but also the total practical experience of the Committee and those consulted. Only a few references have been listed and are intended to represent or amplify certain issues because a complete bibliography of electromyography would occupy several hundred pages.

The Problem

It is axiomatic that all researchers in any scientific area should be able to communicate with clarity the results of their work. The area of electromyography is one where inconsistent and erroneous terms and units are the rule rather than the exception. Even veteran researchers are continuing to contribute to the confusion. The research in many major papers cannot be replicated because of lack of detail on the protocol, recording

*Reprinted with permission of the International Society of Electrophysiological Kinesiology.

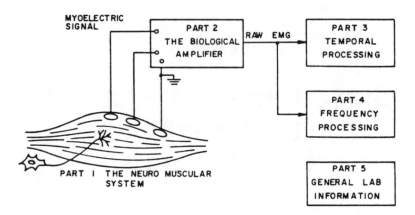

Figure C.1   Schematic outline of scope of report.

equipment, or processing technique. For example, the term integrated EMG (IEMG) has been used to describe at least 4 different processing techniques, and the units employed can be mV, mV/sec, mV • sec, or just arbitrary units! No wonder there are conflicts and misunderstandings.

Form of Report

The report concentrates on four major aspects of the myoelectric signal and its subsequent recording and processing. Figure 1 shows the breakdown of the report: Part I—The Neuromuscular Domain, Part II—The Recording System, Part III—Temporal Processing, and Part IV—Frequency Processing. In addition, the Committee presents a Part V—General Experimental Details, which outlines important kinesiological and experimental information that should be reported. References made to the literature are by no means complete, rather they are cited as examples of erroneous or anomalous reporting. Finally, a checklist is given to summarize the recommendations of the Committee.

Part I: Terminology Applied to the Neuromuscular Unit

References: DeLuca, 1979; Buchthal and Schmalbruck, 1980.

α *motoneuron*—is the neural structure whose cell body is located in the anterior horn of the spinal cord and through its relatively large diameter axon and terminal branches innervates a group of muscle fibers.

motor unit (MU)—is the term used to describe the single smallest controllable muscular unit. The motor unit consists of a single α motoneuron, its neuromuscular junction, and the muscle fibers it innervates (as few as 3, as many as 2000).

muscle fiber action potential or motor action potential (MAP)—is the name given to the detected waveform resulting from the depolarization wave as it propagates in both directions along each muscle fiber from its motor end plate. Without the use of special micro techniques it is generally not possible to isolate an individual MAP.

motor unit action potential (MUAP)—is the name given to the detected waveform consisting of the spatio-temporal summation of individual muscle fiber action potentials originating from muscle fibers in the vicinity of a given electrode or electrode pair. Its shape is a function of electrode type (recording contact area, inter-wire spacing, material, etc.), the location of the electrode with respect to the fibers of the active motor unit, the electrochemical properties of the muscle and connective tissue and the electrical characteristics of the recording equipment. A MUAP detected by a surface electrode will be quite different from the MUAP detected by an indwelling electrode within the muscle tissue. Each motor unit will generally produce a MUAP of characteristic shape and amplitude, as long as the geometric relationship between the electrode and active motor unit remains constant. However, when the MUAP consists of less than about five MAPs the waveform may vary randomly due to the ''jitter'' phenomenon of the neuromuscular junction. A given electrode will record the MUAPs of all active motor units within its pick-up area.

motor unit action potential train (MUAPT)—is the name given to a repetitive sequence of MUAPs from a given motor unit.

inter pulse interval (IPI)—is the time between adjacent discharges of a motor unit. The IPI depends on the level and duration of a contraction and even at an attempted constant tension the IPI is irregular. Its variation is conveniently seen in an IPI histogram.

motor unit firing rate—is the average firing rate of a motor unit over a given period of time. When a motor unit is first recruited it fires at an initial rate and generally increases as the muscle tension increases. Meaningful estimates of average firing rates should be calculated over at least six consecutive IPIs.

synchronization—is the term to describe the tendency for a motor unit to discharge at or near the time that another motor unit discharges. It therefore describes the interdependence or entrainment of two or more motor units.

myoelectric signal—is the name given to the total signal seen at an electrode or differentially between two electrodes. It is the algebraic summation of all MUAPTs from all active motor units within the pick-up area of those electrodes. The myoelectric signal must be amplified before it can be recorded (when it is called an electromyogram).

Part II: The Recording System

INTRODUCTION

With respect to recording electromyographic signals the most important property is the distribution of signal energy in the signal frequency band. The signal frequency spectrum picked up by electrodes depends on:

(a) the type of muscle fiber since the dynamic course of depolarization/repolarization is specific to the muscles (e.g., heart muscle cells, skeletal muscle or smooth muscle cells),
(b) the characteristics of the volume conductor: the electrical field is influenced by the shape, conductivity, and permitivity of tissues and the shape of the boundaries,
(c) the location and physical structure of the electrodes, especially the distance from the cell surface.

Theoretically, the signal source frequency can only be determined by microelectrode techniques at the cellular level. In practice different types of macro-electrodes are utilized: (a) needle electrodes, (b) wire electrodes, (c) surface electrodes. Needle and wire electrodes are invasive, surface electrodes are non-invasive. In clinical diagnosis, needle and wire electrodes are indispensible but the progress in surface electrode methodology has progressed very rapidly mainly because of its wide use. Unfortunately, there are many difficulties which have to be taken into account, and which are now discussed in more detail.

THE PROBLEM

For surface electrode recording, two aspects have to be considered: (1) The electrophysiological sources within the body as a volume conductor, resulting in an electrical field at the skin surface (the upper boundary of volume). Each motor unit contributes independently of each other, and the separation of each of these different sources is increasingly difficult as their distance to the electrode increases. (2) The detection of electrophysiological signals at the skin surface has to take into account the electrical

Table C.1

Signal	Amplitude Range, mV	Signal Frequency Range, Hz	Electrode Type
Indwelling EMG	0.05 - 5	0.1 - 10,000	Needle/Wire
Surface EMG	0.01 - 5	1 - 3,000	Surface
Nerve Potentials	0.005 - 5	0.1 - 10,000	Needle/Wire

properties of the skin, the electrodes, as well as the signal characteristics. The distortion and the disturbances can be reduced by a proper design.

Typical amplitude and frequency range of the signals in question are shown in Table 1. However, the actual ranges depend greatly on the electrode used.

a. Surface electromyography.   The electrodes are electrically coupled to the motor action potentials propagating within the muscle tissue. The stages of this coupling are depicted in Figure 2. These different stages are considered separately and their properties related in order to find out which are first order effects and which can be neglected; please consider Figure 3.

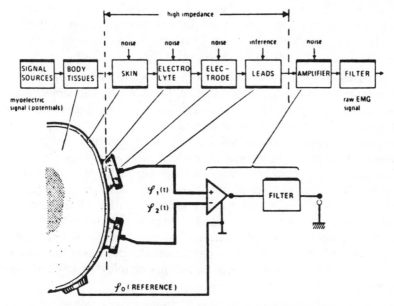

Figure C.2 Measuring set up for surface electromyography.

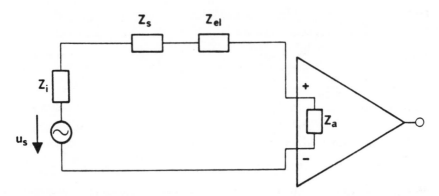

Figure C.3 Simplified circuit with lumped elements describing the most important electrical properties. Z_s = complex skin resistance, Z_{el} = complex resistance of electrodes and electrode/electrode transition, Z_a = complex input resistance of the amplifier, Z_i = complex resistance of the body tissues.

Signal source and body tissues. Within the body a relatively high conductance exists due to the concentration of freely moving ions. The specific resistance is, in the signal frequency band up to 1 KHz, ohmic, and in the order of magnitude of 100-1000 ohm • cm; this value depends on the nature of the tissue in consideration (fat, lung, blood, human trunk). At about 1 KHz the capacitive current and the resistive current are of equal value. Therefore, when using needle or wire electrodes the input impedance of the amplifier should be not less than 1 Megohm, if signal frequencies above 2 KHz have to be detected.

Skin resistance. The resistance of the unprepared skin is complex and varies over a wide range dependent on (a) skin site, (b) subject and (c) time and (d) skin preparation. In worst cases we see values up to several megohms at low frequencies. In order to minimize the influence of this complex resistance on the signal, high input resistance amplifiers can be achieved very easily by means of modern FET-technology.

In most existing instrumentation an input impedance of 10 Megohms or even 1 Megohm is common, thus the skin has to be prepared (rubbed, abraded) until the resistance is down to less than 100 KΩ or even 10 KΩ respectively. Of course, then the impedance between the electrodes should be measured over the whole frequency band. However, the use of a high performance amplifier eliminates the preparation of the skin and the need to check the resistance, thus simplifying the measuring procedure.

Electrode, electrolyte and transition. The electrode resistance and the electrode/electrolyte transition are dependent on the electrode material and the electrolyte (paste or cream) in use. Here not only the electrical but also the mechanical and physiological properties have to be taken into account. Low polarization voltage is observed at Ag-AgCl-Electrodes; unfortunately the Ag-content varies dependent on the manufacturer resulting in differing properties. Stainless steel electrodes are adequate when using them on unprepared skin and for a frequency of above 10 Hz. Long term stability is excellent with black platina.

The electrode and electrode/electrolyte transition can be neglected with respect to the unprepared skin resistance over the entire frequency range; both have similar electrical characteristics. The impedance of both unprepared and prepared skin can be neglected as long as the input impedance of the amplifier is sufficiently high (at least 100 times the skin impedance).

The amplifier.   Modern technology has resulted in amplifier specifications to overcome the measuring problems. However, old instrumentation gives rise to problems of input impedance, input current and noise. The desired and recommended specifications for newly designed amplifiers are as follows:

CMRR > 90 dB

Input resistance > 10^{10} ohms for dc coupled; > 10^8 ohms at 100 Hz for ac coupled.

Input current < 50 nA for directly coupled amplifiers

Noise level < 5 μVrms with a source resistance of 100 KΩ and a frequency bandwidth from 0.1-1000 Hz.

The low input current is to be desired because of artifacts which may be caused by modulation of the skin resistance. It is known that the value Z_s (Figure 3) varies with mechanical pressure. Time varying pressure occurs when movement is induced to the electrodes via cable motion. With a change ΔZ_s = 50 KΩ and an input current of 50 nA the generated voltage is 2.5 mV.

In addition, pressure applied to the skin produces an artifact voltage which cannot be separated from the signal voltage, except by high pass filtering above the frequency of the movement artifact (about 10 Hz). In a recently performed study (Silny et al., 1979) on cable properties some cables produced movement artifacts of several millivolts, even when using ''special ECG cable.'' There are cable types now available which produce 100 times less voltage artifact than other cables.

Regarding the noise, the amplifier must not be tested with a short circuit at the input since the amplifier noise is insignificant compared to when using a high resistance source. Therefore, a high resistance test circuit has to be used when specifying the relevant amplifier noise. Of course, the noise situation is improved when the skin resistance has been reduced by skin preparation. Then an amplifier can be used which is of lower input impedance while the current noise becomes less important. Also, a reduction of signal frequency bandwidth reduces the noise level, and such a reduction should be done whenever possible.

b. Wire and needle electrodes.   When using needle and wire electrodes the skin resistance will not impair the signal acquisition as long as an amplifier has a 10 MΩ input impedance. Even fine wire electrodes with a small area of active tip show a relatively low impedance. The properties are mainly defined by the electrode-electrolyte transition and if there are no noise problems in specific applications, one can use the same amplifier as in surface electromyographs.

SUMMARY AND RECOMMENDATIONS

a. Amplifier:

(i) The frequency range of the amplifier channel should be chosen according to Table 1. If in surface electromyography the lower cut-off frequency has been selected to be 20 Hz for suppression of movement artifacts it has to be reported.

Report: upper cut-off frequency
       lower cut-off frequency
       type of filter, slope

(ii) If a DC coupled amplifier is used, a higher input impedance and low input current are desired. AC coupling by a capacitor in each of the two differential electrode leads is commonly used but may give rise to large movement artifacts and polarization voltages if the input impedance is too high. Thus a somewhat lower input impedance is suggested.

Report: input impedance
       input current, if dc coupled
       noise with 100 KΩ at the input, $1<f<1000$ Hz
       CMRR

b. Electrodes:

Report: type
       spacing between recording contacts

material
stability, if important
off set voltage, if important

c. Skin:

Report: site
   complex resistance in the whole signal frequency range
      if a low resistance input amplifier is used
   preparation of skin

d. Electrode paste:

Report: type
   manufacturer
   electrochemical properties

Note #1: New instrumentation should be battery operated, at least in the first differential amplifier stage. This will result in a marked suppression of hum interference and when coupled to a computer, or other recording equipment the necessary isolation is achieved.

Note #2: The amplifier can be miniaturized and attached close to the electrodes. The shorter the electrode leads the smaller the picked up disturbances (hum and other interferences). In addition, the CMRR value is not decreased by unnecessary unsymmetries.

Note #3: The best procedure for adjusting the filter characteristics of the complete channel is to have the frequency band unrestricted, perform a frequency analysis and then adapt the filter bandwidth to the signal bandwidth.

Part III: Temporal Processing

RAW EMG

Visual inspection of the raw EMG is the most common way of examining muscle activity as it changes with time. Correlation of such phasic activity with other biomechanical variables (joint angles, acceleration, moments of force, etc.) or physiological variables has added to the understanding of normal muscle function as well as special motor functions in pathologies, in ergonomic situations and in athletic events. The amplitude of the raw EMG when reported should be that seen at the electrodes, in mV or μV, and should not reflect the gain of any amplifiers in the recording system.

DETECTORS

The quantification of the "amount of activity" is necessary so that researchers can compare results, not only within their own laboratories, but between laboratories. It is important to know not only when a muscle turns on or off, but how much it is on at all times during a given contraction. The basis for most of this quantification comes from a detector. A linear detector is nothing more than a full-wave rectifier which reverses the sign of all negative voltages and yields the absolute value of the raw EMG. Non-linear detectors can also be used. For example, a square law detector is the basis of the root mean square (rms) value of the EMG. The important point is that the details of the detector must always be reported because the results of subsequent processing and conclusions regarding muscle function are strongly influenced by the detector (Kadefors, 1973).

TYPES OF AVERAGES

(a) Average or mean.   The mean EMG is the time average of the full-wave rectified EMG over a specified period of time. It is therefore, important for the researcher to specify the time over which the average was taken. Is it the duration of the contraction, the stride period, or the total exercise period? The mean value should be reported in mV (or μV), and for a period of (t_2-t_1) seconds,

$$\text{Mean} = \frac{1}{(t_2-t_1)} \int_{t_1}^{t_2} \left| \text{EMG} \right| \ dt \qquad \text{mV}$$

(b) Moving averages.   It is often valuable to see how the EMG activity changes with time over the period of contraction, and a moving average is usually the answer. Several common processing techniques are employed with the detected signal (usually full-wave rectified). All moving averages are in mV or μV.

The most common is a low-pass filter, which follows the peaks and valleys of the full-wave rectified signal. Thus the characteristics of the filter should be specified (i.e., 2nd order Butterworth low-pass filter with cutoff at 6 Hz). It is somewhat confusing and meaningless to report the average time constant of the filter especially if a 2nd order or higher order filter is used. The combination of a full-wave rectifier followed by a low-pass filter is commonly referred to as a linear envelope detector.

With the advent of digital filtering the processing of the EMG can be processed many novel ways. Analog low-pass filters, for example, introduce a phase lag in the output, whereas digital filters can have zero phase shift (by first filtering in the positive direction of time, then refiltering in the negative direction of time). If such processing is used, the net filter characteristics should be quoted (i.e., 4th order zero-lag, low pass Butterworth filter with cut-off at 10 Hz).

Probably the most common digital moving-average type is realized by a "window" which calculates the mean of the detected EMG over the period of the window. As the window moves forward in time a new average is calculated. It can be expressed as follows:

$$\text{Window Average (t)} = \frac{1}{T} \int_{t-T/2}^{t+T/2} |EMG| \; dt \qquad mV$$

Its value is in mV, and all that is needed is to specify the window width, T. Normally the average is calculated for the middle of the window because it does not introduce a lag in its output. However, if the moving average is calculated only for past history the expression becomes:

$$\text{Window Average (t)} = \frac{1}{T} \int_{0}^{t+T} |EMG| \; dt \qquad mV$$

Such an average introduces a phase lag which increases with T, thus if this type is used T should be clearly indicated. Other special forms of weighting (exponential, triangular, etc.) should be clearly described.

(c) Ensemble average.   In any repetitive movement or evoked response it is often important to get the average pattern of EMG activity. An ensemble average is accomplished digitally in a general purpose computer or in special computers of average transients (C.A.T.). With evoked stimuli it is often possible to average the resultant compound action potentials. The time-averaged waveform has an amplitude in mV, and the number of averages is important to report. Also, the standard error at each point in time may be important. The expression for N time-averaged waveforms at any time t is:

$$EMG \; (t) = \frac{1}{N} \sum_{i=1}^{N} |EMG_i| \; (t) \qquad mV$$

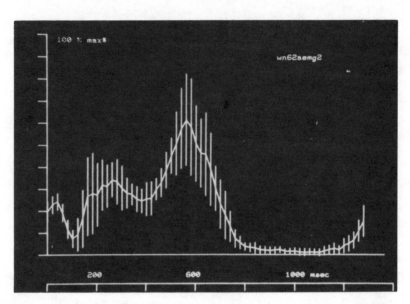

Figure C.4   Average of linear envelope of soleus muscle over 10 walking strides. Contraction was normalized to 100% MVC, and standard deviation at each point in time is shown by vertical bars.

where EMG_i is the ith repetition of the EMG waveform to be averaged. An example of such an averaged waveform is presented in Figure 4; the linear envelope of the soleus muscle was averaged over 10 strides. A complete stride is shown; the amplitude would normally be in mV or μV, but here it is reported as a percentage of the EMG at 100% maximum voluntary contraction. There is no consensus at present as to standard methods of eliciting a maximum contraction because of variations in muscle length with different limb positions and the inhibitary influences present in agonist and antagonist muscle groups. However, such normalization techniques are indispensible for comparisons between different subjects and for retrials on the same subject.

Integrated EMG.   Probably the most widely used (and abused) term in electromyography today is integrated EMG (IEMG). Probably the first use of the term was by Inman and co-workers (1952) when they described a waveform which followed the rise and fall in tension in the muscle. The circuit they employed was a linear envelope detector, not an integrator. The correct interpretation of integration is purely mathematical, and means the "area under the curve." The units of IEMG have also been widely abused. For example, Komi (1973) reports IEMG in mV/s, and in 1976 scales the IEMG in mV. The correct units are mV • s or μV • s. It is suspected that many of these researchers who report IEMG in mV are

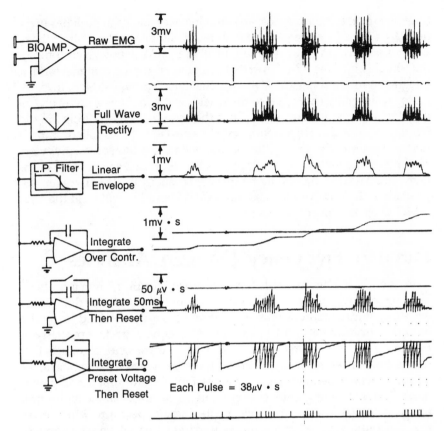

Figure C.5 Examples of several common types of temporal processing of the EMG.

really reporting the average over an unspecified period of time and not an integration over that period.

There are many versions of integrated EMG's. Figure 5 shows a diagram of 3 common versions, plus the linear envelope signal that is so often misrepresented as an IEMG. The raw and full-wave rectified signals are shown for several bursts of activity and have their amplitudes reported in mV. The linear envelope as shown employed a second order low-pass filter with cut-off at 6 Hz, its amplitude also appears in mV.

The simplest form of integration starts at some preset time and continues during the total time of muscle activity. Over any desired period of time the IEMG can be seen in mV • s. A second form of integrator involves a resetting of the integrated signal to zero at regular intervals of time (usually from 50 to 200 ms), and the time should be specified. Such a scheme yields a series of peaks which represent the trend of the EMG amplitude with time; in effect, something close to a moving average. Each peak has units of mV • s (or μV • s because the integrated value over these short times will not exceed 1 mV • s). The sum of all the peaks in any given contraction should equal the IEMG over that contraction. A third common form of integration uses a voltage level reset. If the muscle activity is high, the integrator will rapidly charge up to the reset level, and if low activity occurs it will take longer to reach reset. Thus the activity level is reflected in the frequency of resets. High frequency of resets (sometimes called "pips") means high muscle activity, low frequency means low level activity, as seen by the lower trace of Figure 5. Each reset represents a value of integrated EMG and this should be specified (usually in μV • s). Again, the product of the number of resets times this calibration will yield the total IEMG over any given period of time.

Part IV: Frequency Domain Analyses

Frequency domain methods have been used for more than a century. They have proven a powerful tool in that solutions to a linear differential equation of a function of time, say, are most easily obtained using the Fourier transform or Laplace transform. A second attractive property of Fourier transforms of functions of time (such as myoelectric signals) is that the function is described as a function of frequency (not to be confused, for example, with repetition rate of a succession of motor unit action potentials). A signal having finite energy content, such as a single motor unit action potential, can be described by its energy spectrum, which gives the distribution of energy as a function of frequency. A signal having infinite energy content, such as a hypothetical infinite succession of action potentials or an infinitely long interference pattern of the activity of several motor units, can similarly be characterized by its power spectrum. In practical work, a time-limited stretch of data is often regarded as periodically repeated (from long before Moses till after the end of time and thus is for infinite duration). The concept of power spectrum is consequently used unless the data is explicitly time-limited as for instance when stress is on one action potential. The square-root of the power spectrum and the square-root of the energy spectrum are both referred to as the amplitude spectrum. Figure 6 shows examples of two motor-unit potentials (modelled as differentiated Gauss pulses) with their amplitude and energy spectra.

UNITS OF MEASUREMENT

Frequency is measured in Hz (Hertz), formerly in English literature in cycles per second. The name energy spectrum was originally devised for

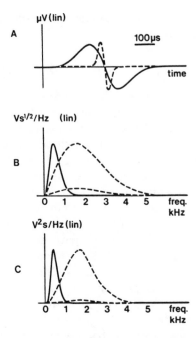

Figure C.6 (a) Two examples of action potentials, modelled as differentiated Gauss pulses. The duration of the wider potential is four times that of the shorter one. (b) Amplitude spectra of the two pulses. (c) Energy spectra of the two pulses. The lower dashed curves indicate the factual spectra of the short action potential; the upper dashed curves have been normalized to the same spectral peak magnitudes as those of the wide action potential. Linear scales, arbitrary magnitudes.

measures of electrical energy decomposed as a function of frequency. The unit for this quantity is joules[1] per hertz, abbreviated J/Hz or J Hz^{-1}. Similarly, the unit of the power spectrum is watts per hertz, W/Hz. Over the years, as frequency domain methods have become used more and more in the study of problems not related directly to energy and power, the names energy spectrum and power spectrum have been given a wider meaning. Thus, the units applied are not restricted to what is said above. Consider the example of EMG. The unit of power spectrum is the square of the unit of the amplitude of the myoelectric signal per hertz, that is volt squared per Hz, V^2/Hz. The unit of the power spectrum of the distance from earth to the moon (measured as a function of time) similarly is meters squared per Hz, m^2/Hz. The unit of the energy spectrum of an action potential is V^{2}s/Hz. The unit for the amplitude spectrum of EMG is thus

---

[1]One joule was formerly referred to as one wattsecond.

either V/Hz, if one starts from the power spectrum, or Vs$^{1/2}$/Hz, if one starts from the energy spectrum.

LOGARITHMIC SCALES AND NORMALIZATION

In visualizing spectra in graphs, valuable information is often lost due to the limited dynamic range of linear scales. For instance, if the maximum value of a power spectrum is 100 V^2/Hz and interesting phenomena occur at a level of 1 or 0.1 V^2/Hz, they will obviously be lost to the eye if the plot is on linear scales. The cure is to plot the spectrum on double logarithm scales or on linear-logarithmic scales. In order to take the logarithm of a quantity, it is necessary that the quantity have no dimension. For example, the logarithm of 2 volts is not defined. By normalizing 2 volts, by referring it to for instance 1 volt (the unit of measurement), one obtains the dimensionless quantity 2, which has a logarithm. The level of reference may be chosen freely as long as it has the same unit as the variable of interest. The concept of decibel,[2] dB, is used for logarithmically scaled power, energy, and amplitude spectra. One may thus plot a spectrum on log-lin scales in the form of "decibels vs logarithmically scaled frequency." Figure 7 illustrates the effect of logarithmizing the spectra of Figure 6. Caution should be exerted to ensure that the plot should not extend below the noise level of the system.

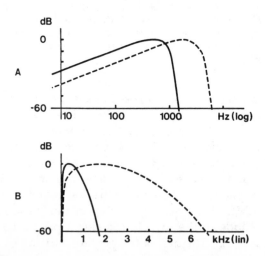

Figure C.7 Effect of logarithmizing the spectra of Figure C.6. (a) Double logarithmic, and (b) log/lin scales. The spectra have been normalized to the same peak magnitude.

---

[2]The decibel concept is, to be strict, linked with power ratios; the gain in decibels of a system equals ten times the base ten logarithm of the ratio of output to input power.

DISCRETE PARAMETERS OF SPECTRA

To report research results as functions of one variable is difficult. Among the problems is the question of proper statistical evaluation. One solution is to reduce the information to what is carried by discrete parameters. There is of course a large number of such parameters (this is the very cause of the problem). A few that have been used in the analysis of EMG will be mentioned here.

Figure 8(a) shows an example of a spectrum plotted on logarithmic scales. In the case of a smooth and unimodal spectrum like the one shown, one can easily find the upper and lower 3-dB frequencies, defined by the frequencies at which the spectrum has fallen 3 dB from its maximum value. The 3-dB bandwidth is defined at the difference between the upper and lower 3-dB frequencies (fb and fa, respectively), and the center frequency fc is given by the geometric mean of the 3-dB frequencies. A 3-dB drop is equivalent to a decrease by 50% in a linear scale representation of the power spectrum (see Figure 8(b)), and are therefore referred to as half-power frequencies.

In Figure 8(a) is shown a piecewise linear approximation, known as the asymptotic Bode diagram. This asymptotic diagram is entirely defined

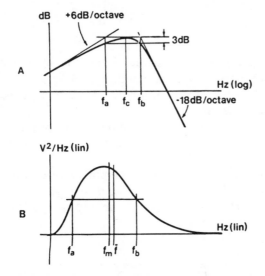

Figure C.8 (a) An example of a power spectrum, with high-frequency and low-frequency asymptots indicated, and 3-dB limits given. Double logarithmic scales. (b) Same power spectrum as above, with linear scales, and with some parameters of interest given; fm and f denote the median and the mean frequencies, respectively. The locations are approximate. In principle, the areas under the curve on both sides of fm are identical, whereas f denotes the frequency where the area under the curve would balance if cut out with scissors.

by the slopes of the lines, the frequencies where the slope changes, the breakpoints, and a scale factor.

The variables discussed so far are commonly used in engineering sciences. Now we will discuss several parameters that have parallels in statistics. In order to do so, the concepts of spectral movements will first be defined. The spectral moment of order n is given by:

$$m_n = \int_0^\infty f^n W(f)\, df$$

where f is frequency and W is the power or energy spectrum.

The mean frequency, f, is the ratio between the spectral moments or orders one and zero (similar to the mean value in statistics). Thus:

$$\bar{f} = \frac{m_1}{m_0} \qquad \frac{\displaystyle\int_0^f f\, W(f)\, df}{\displaystyle\int_0^f W(f)\, df} \qquad Hz$$

The statistical bandwidth is the square-root of the difference between the ratio of the moment of order two to that of order zero and the square of the mean frequency (cf. the standard deviation in statistics). Rice has shown that, for Gaussian noise, the intensity of zero crossings equals the square-root of the ratio between the moments of orders two and zero, and the intensity of turning points equals the ratio between the fourth and second order moments.

The frequency at the maximum of the power spectrum may be called the mode (most probable frequency), and the median frequency fm is the frequency which divides the spectrum into two parts of equal power (energy), and is defined by:

$$\int_0^{fm} W(f)\, df = \int_{fm}^\infty W(f)\, df$$

All these parameters, and several not mentioned here, have been used in reports on EMG-research results. The parameters have different properties as they emphasize different aspects of the spectrum. It would be premature to recommend the use of any specific subset, if such a recommendation should ever be made. It is, however, important to know of the various possibilities, and to be familiar with the properties of the parameters.

SPECTRAL ESTIMATION

Integrals over an infinite time period appear in the mathematical definition of the power spectrum of a noise signal. For obvious reasons then, spectra can never be evaluated exactly; rather any spectrum obtained is an estimate of the mathematical concept. The use of finite stretches of raw EMG data introduces estimation errors. These errors are often summarized as the bias of the estimate, the systematic error, and the variance of the estimate, the statistical uncertainty. Methods employed to reduce these errors include windowing of the raw data, averaging of successive spectral estimates and smoothing of spectral estimates. In reporting results based on spectral analysis, it is important to state the estimation procedure and, if possible, give figures on the bias and the variance of the final estimate. It is important also to report questions pertinent to other sources of errors. In particular, one should give some indication on the noise level of the experimental setup, and state the sampling rate if digital methods are used. The possibility of excessive line interference is easily checked by visual inspection of the spectra obtained.

Part V: General Experimental and Kinesiological Information

One major drawback which prevents a full understanding, comparison or replication of any EMG research is inadequate detail of the protocol itself especially related to the anatomy, physiology and biomechanics of the neuromusculo-skeletal system under test.

TYPES OF CONTRACTION

1. Isometric—muscle has an average fixed length or joint is at a fixed angle (specify length or angle).
2. Isotonic—a contraction which produces an average constant force or, for in vivo contractions at an average constant moment (torque) (specify force (N) or moment (N • m)). Remember, that lifting or lowering a mass is not isotonic unless it is moving at a constant velocity.

3. Isokinetic—muscle is contracting at a constant linear velocity, or constant angular velocity (specify velocity (m/s) or angular velocity (rad/s)).
4. Concentric—muscle is shortening under tension.
5. Eccentric—muscle is lengthening under tension.

ASSOCIATED BIOMECHANICAL TERMS

1. Mechanical Energy—is the energy state of any limb segment or total body system at an instant in time. It is measured in joules (J).
2. Mechanical Power—is the rate of doing work or rate of change of energy at an instant of time. It is measured in watts (W).
3. Mechanical Work—is the time integral of the mechanical power over a specified period of time. It is also equal to the change in energy of a system (segment or total body) over that same period of time. It is measured in joules (J).
4. Positive Work—is the work done by concentrically contracting muscles. Thus the time integral of mechanical power over a specified time is positive, or the net change in energy of the system is also positive.
5. Negative Work—is the work done by an eccentrically contracting muscle. Thus the time integral of mechanical power over the specified time is negative, or the net change in energy of the system is negative.
6. Moment of Force (Torque)—Product of a force and lever arm distance about a centre of rotation (usually a joint centre). The unit is Newton-meters (N • m).
7. Impulse—is the time integral of a force or moment curve, and is usually employed in ballistic movements to reflect changes in momentum of the associated limbs. Linear impulse is quantified in N • s, angular impulses in N • m • s. The impulse is a prerequisite to calculation of average force or moment over a given period of time.

ELECTRODE AND ANATOMICAL DETAILS

The type and position of the electrodes must be reported. If indwelling electrodes are used additional information is necessary (needle, wire, unipolar, bipolar, depth of electrode, etc.). If there are problems of cross-talk the exact positioning of electrodes is necessary along with details of any precautionary tests that were done to ensure minimal cross-talk. If cocontractions can nullify or modify your results some evidence is necessary to demonstrate that the antagonistic activity was negligible.

It is now quite common to quantify an EMG amplitude as a percentage of maximum voluntary contraction (MVC). The details as to how these were elicited are important. Also, the position of the body, adjacent limbs, etc., need to be described.

If electrical stimulation is being done, additional electrode data are necessary: position of anode and cathode, surface area of contact or, in case of indwelling electrodes, details of the exposed conductive surface. The strength, duration and frequency of the stimulating pulses is mandatory, and remember that the strength is usually in current units (ma) rather than voltage, because the net depolarization is a function of current leaving the electrodes. Without a knowledge of skin/electrode impedance, the voltage information is not too meaningful. Thus with a constant voltage stimulation it is important to monitor and report the current pulse waveform.

GENERAL SUBJECT INFORMATION

In any population study it is often relevant to give details of age, sex, height, and weight of normals that may sometimes influence the results of certain experiments. Also, in conditions of fatigue or special training appropriate measures should be specified. For athletic or ergonomic tasks the researcher must give sufficient information to ensure that other centres could replicate his experiments. In the assessment of pathological movements certain clinical and medical history details of each patient may be necessary (i.e., level of lesion, number of months since stroke, type of prosthesis).

References

Buchthal, F. and Schmalbruch, H. Motor unit of mammalian muscle. Physiol. Rev. 60:90-142, 1980.

DeLuca, C.J. Physiology and mathematics of myoelectric signals. IEEE Trans. Biomed. Engng. BME—26:313-325, 1979.

Inman, V.T. et al. Relation of human EMG to muscle tension. EEG and Clinical Neurophysiology. 4:187-194, 1952.

Kadefors, R. Myoelectric signal processing as an estimation problem. New Developments in EMG and Clinical Neurophysiology. Vol. 1, 519-532 (Karger, Basel, 1973).

Komi, P.V. and Viitasalo, J.H.T. Signal characteristics of EMG at different levels of muscle tension. Acta Physiol. Scand. 96:267-276, 1976.

Komi, P.V. Relationship between muscle, tension, EMG and velocity of contraction under concentric and eccentric work. New Developments in EMG and Clinical Neurophysiology. Vol. 1, 596-606 (Karger, Basel, 1973).

Silny, J., Hinsen, R., Rau, G., vonEssen, R., Merx, W. and Effert, S. Multiple-electrode measuring system for electrocardiographic evaluation of the course of acute myocardial infarction. Biomedizinische Technik 24:106-112, 1979.

A Checklist of Common Terms

TERMINOLOGY	UNITS	COMMENTS/RECOMMENDATION
Amplifier Gain	ratio or dB	
Input Resistance or Impedance	ohms	10^{10} (resistance) on new dc equipment, 10^8 (impedance) on new ac amplifiers at 100 Hz Min. 100 times skin impedance
Common Mode Rejection Ratio (CMRR)	ratio or dB	90 dB or better
Filter cut-off or Bandwidth	Hz	type and order of filter
EMG (raw signal)	mV	
EMG (average)	mV	specify averaging period
EMG (F.W. Rect.)	mV	
EMG (non-linear detector)	mV	specify non-linearity (i.e. square law)
EMG (linear envelope)	mV	cut-off frequency and type of low-pass filter
Integrated EMG (iEMG)	mV · s	specify integration period
Integrated EMG and Reset every T	mV · s or μV · s	specify T (ms)
Integrated EMG to Threshold and Reset	mV · s or μV · s	specify threshold (mV · s)
Power Spectral Density Function (PSDF)	μV²/Hz	
Mean Spectral Frequency (MSF)	Hz	
Median Frequency	Hz	

Appendix D

Sample Budget

This sample budget is for a filming project to examine 10 different athletes in a typical testing situation. The movement to be examined is planar. Although the test situation is hypothetical, it may have several applications. One assumption in this example is that the computer programs for data reduction and analysis are already in place. In some laboratories, the testing is performed on a cost per subject basis, which will include built-in costs according to the following schedule. The frame rate utilized will be 50 pictures per second (pps), affecting the amount of film used. The faster the frame rate, of course, the more film that is used. The project for the enclosed budget is a simple filming task to determine some kinematic factors during the progression of the athletes. Therefore, the amount is quite minimal. Every project budget should be discussed by both the researcher/tester and the requesting group before the actual work begins. In many instances, the contribution of the personnel can be reduced. However, costs for some personnel may be higher, depending on the specific laboratory used. Again, these costs and all related expenditures for the defined project should be well described and agreed upon by both parties before any work is begun.

If added analysis and the use of other equipment is also required, the costs will necessarily increase. Such items as force platforms, pressure transducers, electrogoniometers, and the associated transmitters, receivers, records, and so on, all increase the cost in terms of equipment, supplies, and personnel. As a final comment, it is always possible to find someone who will do the work you require very cheaply, but you can expect results in line only with what you are willing to pay. As in any purchase, good value does not always mean the cheapest.

Table D.1 Budget for Film Project

Expense item		Cost
Personnel:		
Biomechanist 3 days at $350/day		$1,050.00
Computer technician 5 hr at $25/hr		125.00
Graduate student 50 hr at $10/hr		500.00
Laboratory technician 10 hr at $20/hr		200.00
Secretarial help 10 hr at $8/hr		80.00
	Total personnel	$1,955.00
Supplies:		
Film 10 × 100′ rolls at $40/roll (processing included)		$ 400.00
Photographs, film, slides, and so on (for presentation and publication)		100.00
Photocopying (final report + articles) (approximately 1,000 pages × .08)		80.00
Consumable supplies (paper, typewriter ribbons, correction fluid, pens, pencils, letraset, etc.)		100.00
Laboratory supplies (tape, markers, etc.)		25.00
	Total supplies	$ 705.00
Computer Costs:		
5 hr computer time at $100/hr		$ 500.00
Overhead (50% of total contract):		$1,580.00
Maintenance costs of equipment		
Use of facilities		
Administration costs of contract		
Optional items		
	TOTAL	$4,740.00

References

Abbott, B.C., Bigland, B., & Ritchie, J.M. (1952). The physiological cost of negative work. *Journal of Physiology*, **117**, 380-390.

Amtech-Cook Model no OR6-2 multi-component force and torque measuring platform. (1978). *Newsletter of the Force Platform Group, I.S.B.*, **5**, 35-36.

Amti 6-component biomechanical platforms. (1980). *Newsletter of the Force Platform Group, I.S.B.*, **10**, 14-15.

Andersson, G.B.J., Ortengren, R., & Schultz, A. (1980). Analysis and measurement of the loads on the lumbar spine during work at a table. *Journal of Biomechanics*, **13**, 513-520.

Arcan, M., & Brull, M.A. (1976). A fundamental characteristic of the human body and foot, the foot-ground pressure pattern. *Journal of Biomechanics*, **9**, 453-457.

Atkinson, P.J., & Wheatherell, J.A. (1967). Variation in the density of the femoral diaphysis with age. *The Journal of Bone and Joint Surgery*, **49B**(4), 781-788.

Barter, J.T. (1957). *Estimation of the mass of body segments* (WADC-57-260). Wright-Patterson Air Force Base, OH: Aerospace Medical Research Laboratory.

Bishop, P.J. (1976). Ice hockey helmets: Using a mathematical model of head protection for evaluating standards. *Journal of Safety Research*, **8**, 163-170.

Bishop, P.J. (1977). Comparative impact performance capabilities of ice hockey helmets. *Journal of Safety Research*, **9**, 159-167.

Boccardi, S., Pedotti, A., Rodano, R., & Santambrogio, C. (1981). Evaluation of muscular moments at the lower limb joints by an on-line processing of kinematic data and ground reaction. *Journal of Biomechanics*, **14**, 35-45.

Bodine-Reese, P., & Bone, J.P. (1976). Premotor reaction time component of biceps brachii, brachialis and brachioradialis muscles in varsity versus non-varsity women. In P.V. Komi (Ed.), *Biomechanics V-A*, pp. 96-101. Baltimore: University Park Press.

Bouisset, S., & Pertuzon, E. (1968). Experimental determination of the moment of inertia of limb segments. *Biomechanics I* (pp. 106-109). First International Seminar. Zurich: Karger, Basel.

Burley, L.R. (1944). A study of the reaction time of physically trained men. *Research Quarterly*, 15, 232-239.

Cappozzo, A., Figura, F., & Marchetti, M. (1976). The interplay of muscular and external forces in human ambulation. *Journal of Biomechanics*, 9, 35-43.

Cappozzo, A., Leo, T., & Pedotti, A. (1975). A general computing method for the analysis of human locomotion. *Journal of Biomechanics*, 8, 307-320.

Cavagna, G.A. (1977). Storage and utilization of elastic energy in skeletal muscle. In R.S. Hutton (Ed.), *Exercise and Sport Sciences Reviews Vol. 5* (pp. 89-129). Santa Barbara, CA: J. Publishing Affiliates.

Cavagna, G.A., & Kaneko, M. (1977). Mechanical work and efficiency in level walking and running. *Journal of Physiology*, 268, 467-481.

Cavagna, G.A., Komarck, L., & Mazzoleni, S. (1971). The mechanics of sprint running. *Journal of Physiology*, 217, 709-721.

Cavagna, G.A., & Margaria, R. (1966). Mechanics of walking. *Journal of Applied Physiology*, 21(1), 271-278.

Cavagna, G.A., Saibene, F.P., & Margaria, R. (1963). External work in walking. *Journal of Applied Physiology*, 18, 1-9.

Cavagna, G., Saibene, F.P., & Margaria, R. (1964). Mechanical work in running. *Journal of Applied Physiology*, 19, 249-256.

Cavanagh, P.R., & Gregor, R. (1974). The quick-release method for estimating the moment of inertia of the shank and foot. In R.C. Nelson & C.A. Morehouse (Eds.), *Biomechanics IV* (pp. 524-530). Baltimore: University Park Press.

Cavanagh, P.R., & Gregor, R.J. (1975). Knee joint torque during the swing phase of normal treadmill walking. *Journal of Biomechanics*, 8, 337-344.

Cavanagh, P.R., & Michiyoshi, A. (1980). A technique for the display of pressure distribution beneath the foot. *Journal of Biomechanics*, 13(2), 69-75.

Chaffin, D.B. (1969). A computerized biomechanical model—development of and use in studying gross body actions. *Journal of Biomechanics*, 2, 429-441.

Chao, E.Y. (1978). Experimental methods for biomechanical measurement of joint kinematics. *CRC Handbook of Engineering in Medicine and Biology*, 1B, 385-411.

Chao, E.Y. (1980). Justification of triaxial goniometer for the measurement of joint rotation. *Journal of Biomechanics*, 13, 989-1006.

Clarke, D.H. (1964). The correlation between strength and the rate of tension development of a static muscular contraction. *Internationale Zeitschrift fur Angewandte Physiologie*, 20, 202-206.

Clauser, C.E., McConville, J.T., & Young, J.W. (1969). *Weight, volume and center of mass segments of the human body* (AMRL-TR-69-70). Wright-

Patterson Air Force Base, OH: Aerospace Medical Research Laboratory.

Cleveland, H.G. (1955). *The determination of the center of gravity of segments of the human body.* Unpublished doctoral dissertation, University of California, Los Angeles.

Cohen, H.L., & Brunlik, J. (1976). *Electroneuromyography.* New York: Harper & Row.

Conati, F.C. (1977). *Real-time measurement of three-dimensional multiple rigid body motion.* Unpublished doctoral dissertation, Massachusetts Institute of Technology, Cambridge, MA.

Connolly, K.J. (1970). *Mechanisms of motor skill development.* New York: Academic Press.

Costill, D.L., Daniels, J., Evans, W., Fink, W., Krahenbuhl, G., & Saltin, B. (1976). Skeletal muscle enzymes and fiber composition in male and female track athletes. *Journal of Applied Physiology, 40,* 149-154.

Cousins, S.J. (1975). *A parallelogram chain designed to measure human joint motion.* Unpublished master's thesis, University of British Columbia, Vancouver.

Cureton, T.K. (1951). *Physical fitness of champion athletes.* Urbana, IL: University of Illinois Press.

Dantzig, G.B. (1968). *Linear programming.* New York: McGraw Hill.

Dapena, J. (1981). Simulation of modified human airborne movements. *Journal of Biomechanics, 14,* 81-89.

Dempster, W.T. (1955). *Space requirements for the seated operator* (WADC-TR-55-159). Wright-Patterson Air Force Base, OH: Aerospace Medical Research Laboratory.

Draganich, L.F., Andriacchi, T.P., Strongwater, A.M., & Galante, J.O. (1980). Electronic measurement of instantaneous foot-floor contact patterns during gait. *Journal of Biomechanics, 13,* 875-880.

Drillis, R., & Contini, R. (1966). *Body segment parameters* (1166.03). New York: New York University School of Science and Engineering.

Easton, T.A. (1972). On the normal use of reflexes. *American Scientist, 60,* 591-599.

Edstrom, L. & Ekblom, B. (1972). Differences in sizes of red and white muscle fibers in vastus lateralis of musculus quadriceps femoris of normal individuals and athletes. Relation to physical performance. *Scandinavian Journal of Clinical Laboratory Investigation, 30,* 175-181.

Elftman, H. (1939). Forces and energy changes in the leg during walking. *American Journal of Physiology, 125,* 339-356.

Fenn, W.O. (1930). Frictional and kinetic factors in the work of sprint running. *American Journal of Physiology, 92,* 583-611.

Fidanza, F., & Anderson, J.T. (1953). Density of body fat in a man and other mammals. *Journal of Applied Physiology, 6,* 252-256.

Finley, F.R., Wirta, R.W., & Cody, K.A. (1967). Muscle synergies in motor performance. *Archives of Physical Medicine and Performance*, **49**, 655-660.

Fleury, M., & Lagasse, P.P. (1979). Influence of functional electrical stimulation training on premotor and motor reaction time. *Perceptual and Motor Skills*, **48**, 387-393.

Francis, P.R., & Tipton, C.M. (1969). Influence of a weight training program on quadriceps reflex time. *Medicine and Science in Sports*, **1**, 91-94.

Fukuda, T. (1961). Studies on human dynamic posture from the viewpoint of postural reflexes. *Acta Oto-Laryngolica* (Suppl. 161), 1-52.

Gaesser, G.A., & Brooks, G.A. (1975). Muscular efficiency during steady-rate exercise: Effects of speed and work rate. *Journal of Applied Physiology*, **38**(6), 1132-1139.

Gage, J. (1964). *Accelerographic analysis of human gait*. American Society of Mechanical Engineers Paper No. 64-WA/HUF 08.

Gagnon, M. (1978a). Biomechanical comparison of the standing and kneeling sprint starts. In F. Landry & W.A.R. Orban (Eds.), *Biomechanics of Sports and Kinanthropometry* (pp. 115-122). The International Congress of Physical Activity Sciences, July 1976, Quebec. Miami, FL: Symposia Specialists.

Gagnon, M. (1978b). The use of several force platforms to obtain human kinetic data. *Newsletter of the Force Platform Group, I.S.B.*, **5**, 27-34.

Gagnon, M., & Montpetit, R. (1981). Technological development for the measurement of the center of volume in the human body. *Journal of Biomechanics*, **14**(4), 235-241.

Gagnon, M., & Rodrigue, D. (1979). Determination of physical properties of the forearm by anthropometry, immersion, and photography methods. *Research Quarterly*, **50**(2), 188-198.

Gatev, V. (1972). Role of inhibition in the development of motor coordination in early childhood. *Developmental and Medical Child Neurology*, **14**, 336-341.

Gersten, J.W., Orr, W., Sexton, A.W., & Okin, D. (1969). External work in level walking. *Journal of Applied Physiology*, **26**, 286-289.

Gollnick, P., Armstrong, R., Saubert, C., Piehl, K., & Saltin, B. (1972). Enzyme activity and fiber composition in skeletal muscle of untrained and trained men. *Journal of Applied Physiology*, **33**, 312-319.

Gollnick, P.D., & Karpovitch, P.V. (1964). Electrogoniometric study of locomotion and of some athletic movements. *Research Quarterly*, **35**, 357-369.

Gottlieb, G.L., & Agarwal, G.C. (1972). The role of the myotatic reflex in the voluntary control of movements. *Brain Research*, **40**, 139-143.

Grainger, J., Norman, R., Winter, D., & Bobet, J. (1983). Day-to-day reproducibility of selected biomechanical variables calculated from film data.

In H. Matsui & K. Kobayashi (Eds.), *Biomechanics VIIIB* (pp. 1239-1247). Champaign, IL: Human Kinetics.

Grieve, D.W., Miller, D.I., Mitchelson, D.L., Paul, J.P., & Smith, A.J. (1975). *Techniques for the analysis of human movement* (pp. 69-105). Princeton, NJ: Princeton Book.

Gustafsson, L., & Lanshammar, H. (1977). *ENOCH—an integrated system for measurement and analysis of human gait.* Unpublished doctoral dissertation, Uppsala University, Uppsala, Sweden.

Gutewort, W. (1971). The numerical presentations of the kinematics of human motions. In J. Vredenbregt & J. Wartenweiler (Eds.), *Medicine and Sport, Biomechanics II* (pp. 290-298). Baltimore: University Park Press.

Hamming, R.W. (1977). *Digital filters* (p. 134). Englewood Cliffs, NJ: Prentice-Hall.

Hanavan, E.P. (1964). *A Mathematical model of the human body* (AMRL-TR-64-102). Wright-Patterson Air Force Base, OH: Aerospace Medical Research Laboratories.

Hannah, R., Cousins, S.J., & Foort, J. (1978). The CARS-UBS electrogoniometer—a clinically valuable tool. *Proceedings of the Canadian Medical and Biological Engineering Conference* (pp. 133-144).

Hatze, H. (1975). A new method for the simultaneous measurement of the moment of inertia, the damping coefficient and the location of the centre of mass of a body segment in situ. *European Journal of Applied Physiology,* **34**, 217-225.

Hatze, H. (1980). A mathematical model for the computational determination of parameter values of anthropomorphic segments. *Journal of Biomechanics,* **13**, 833-843.

Hatze, H. (1981). The use of optimally regularized Fourier series for estimating higher order derivatives of noisy biomechanical data. *Journal of Biomechanics,* **14**, 13-18.

Hay, J.G., Wilson, B.D., & Dapena, J. (1976). Identification of the limiting factors in the performance of a basic human movement. In P.V. Komi (Ed.), *Biomechanics V-B.* International Series on Biomechanics (pp. 13-19). Baltimore: University Park Press.

Hayes, K.C. (1972). Jendrassik maneuver facilitation and fractionated patellar reflex times. *Journal of Applied Physiology,* **32**, 290-295.

Hayes, K.C., & Hatze, H. (1977). Passive visco-elastic properties of the structures spanning the human elbow joint. *European Journal of Applied Physiology,* **37**, 265-274.

Hennig, E.M., Cavanagh, P.R., & Macmillan, N.H. (1980). High resolution in-shoe pressure distribution measurements by piezo-electric transducer. *Proceedings of the Special Conference of the Canadian Society for Biomechanics, Human Locomotion I* (pp. 120-121). London, Ontario: Canadian Society for Biomechanics.

Hennig, E.M., & Nicol, K. (1978). Registration methods for time-dependent pressure distribution measurements with mats working as capacitors. In E. Asmussen & K. Jorgensen (Eds.), *Biomechanics VI-A* (pp. 361-367). International Series on Biomechanics, Baltimore: University Park Press.

Hill, A.V. (1940). The dynamic constants of human muscle. *Proceedings of the Royal Society* (B), **128**, 263-274.

Hobart, D.J., Kelley, D.L., & Bradley, L.S. (1975). Modifications occurring during acquisition of a novel throwing task. *American Journal of Physical Medicine*, **54**, 1-24.

Hobart, D.J., & Vorro, J.R. (1974). Electromyographical analysis of intermittent modifications occurring during acquisition of novel throwing skill. In R.C. Nelson & C.A. Morehouse (Eds.), *Biomechanics IV* (pp. 559-566). Baltimore: University Park Press.

Hobart, D.J., Vorro, J.R., & Dotson, C. (1978). Synchronized myoelectric and cinematographic analysis of skill acquisition. *Journal of Human Movement Studies*, **4**, 155-166.

Hoecke, G., & Gruendler, G. (1975). Use of light trace photography in teaching swimming. In J.P. Clarys & L. Lewille (Eds.), *Swimming II* (pp. 194-206). Baltimore: University Park Press.

Jensen, R.K. (1978). Estimation of the biomechanical properties of three body types using a photogrammetric method. *Journal of Biomechanics*, **11**, 349-358.

Kamen, G.P. (1980). *Fractionated reaction and reflex time after fatiguing isometric and isotonic exercise.* Unpublished doctoral dissertation, University of Massachusetts, Amherst.

Kamon, E., & Gormley, J. (1968). Muscular activity pattern for skilled performance and during learning of horizontal bar exercise. *Ergonomics*, **11**, 345-357.

Kaneko, M., & Yamazaki, T. (1978). Internal mechanical work due to velocity changes of the limb in working on a bicycle ergometer. In L. Assmussen & K. Jorgensen (Eds.), *Biomechanics VI-A* (pp. 86-92). Baltimore: University Park Press.

Katch, V.L., Weltman, A., & Gold, E. (1974). Validity of anthropometric measurements and the segment-zone method for estimating segmental and total body volume. *Medicine and Science in Sports*, **6**(2), 271-276.

Kato, M. (1960). The conduction velocity of the ulnar nerve and the spinal reflex time measured by means of the H wave in average adults and athletes. *Tohoku Journal of Experimental Medicine*, **73**, 74-85.

Keller, L.F. (1942). The relationship of "quickness of bodily movement" to athletic success. *Research Quarterly*, **13**, 146-155.

Kinzel, G.L., (1978). Kistler Type 9281 All multicomponent measuring platform for biomechanics and industry. *Newsletter of the Force Platform Group, I.S.B.*, **5**, 37-39.

Kinzel, G.L., Hillberry, B.M., Hall, A.S., Jr., Sickle, V., & Harvey, W.M. (1972). Measurement of the total motion between two body segments. *Journal of Biomechanics*, **5**, 283-293.

Klissouras, V., & Karpovitch, P.V. (1967). Electrogoniometric study of jumping events. *Research Quarterly*, **38**, 41-47.

Knapp, B.N. (1961). Simple reaction times of selected top-class sportsmen and research students. *Research Quarterly*, **32**, 409-411.

Komarek, L. (1968). Biomechanics of training of simple rhythmic efforts. In J. Vredenbregt & J. Wartenweiler (Eds.), *Biomechanics I* (pp. 209-212). Basel: S. Karger.

Kroll, W., & Clarkson, P.M. (1978). Fractionated reflex time, resisted and unresisted fractionated reaction time under normal and fatigued conditions. In D.M. Landers & R.W. Christina (Eds.), *Psychology of Motor Behavior and Sport 1977* (pp. 106-129). Champaign, IL: Human Kinetics.

Kroll, W., & Morris, A.F. (1976). Use of the electromyograph in fractionated reflex and reaction time experimentation. *Journal of Electro-Physiological Techniques*, **5**, 38-41.

Kulwicki, P.V., Schlei, E.J., & Vergamini, P.L. (1962). *Weightless man: Self-rotation techniques* (AMRL-TR-62-129). Wright-Patterson Air Force Base, OH: Aerospace Medical Research Laboratories.

Lagasse, P.P. (1979). Prediction of maximum speed of human movement by two selected muscular coordination mechanisms and by maximum static strength. *Perceptual and Motor Skills*, **49**, 151-161.

Lagasse, P.P., Dion, D., Rouillard, C., & Normand, M.C. (1981). *Prediction of diving performance* (Report). Quebec: Canadian Amateur Diving Association.

Lamoreaux, L.W. (1971). Kinematic measurements in the study of human walking. *Bulletin of Prosthesis Research*, **3**, 10-15.

Lautenbach, R., & Tuttle, W.W. (1932). The relationship between reflex time and running events in track. *Research Quarterly*, **3**, 138-143.

Lees, A. (1980). An optimized film analysis method based on finite difference techniques. *Journal of Human Movement Studies*, **6**, 165-180.

Leider, M., & Buncke, C.M. (1954). Physical dimensions of the skin. *Archives of Dermatology and Syphilology*, **69**, 563-569.

Le Veau, B. (1977). *Williams and Lissner: Biomechanics of human motion.* Toronto: W.B. Saunders.

Lindahl, O., & Lindgren, A.G.H. (1967). Cortic 1 bone in man. II. Variation in tensile strength with age and sex. *Acta Orthopaedica Scandinavia*, **38**, 141-147.

Lindholm, L.E. (1974). An optoelectronic instrument for remote on-line movement monitoring. In R.C. Nelson & C.A. Morehouse (Eds.), *Biomechanics IV* (pp. 510-512). Baltimore: University Park Press.

Little, M.J., & Jessup, G.T. (1977). Determining limb volume by a point-gauge, water-displacement technique. *Research Quarterly*, **48**(1), 239-243.

MacDougall, J.D., Wenger, H.A., & Green, H.J. (1982). *Physiological testing of the elite athlete*. Ottawa: Canadian Association of Sport Sciences.

Maier, I. (1968). Measurement apparatus and analysis methods of the biomotor process of sports movements. In *Medicine and Sport, Biomechanics I* (pp. 96-101). Baltimore: University Park Press.

Margaria, R. (1968). Positive and negative work performances and their efficiencies in human locomotion. *Internationale Zeitschrift fur Angewandte. Physiologie einschlie Blich Arbeitsphysiologie*, **25**, 339-351.

Margaria, R., Cerretelli, P., & Sassi, G. (1963). Energy cost of running. *Journal of Applied Physiology*, **18**(2), 367-370.

Martin, T.P., & Pongratz, M.B. (1974). Validation of a mathematical model for correction of photographic perspective error. In R.C. Nelson & C.A. Morehouse (Eds.), *Biomechanics IV* (pp. 469-475). Baltimore: University Park Press.

McNeill, T., Warwick, D., Andersson, G., & Schultz, A. (1980). Trunk strength in attempted flexion, extension, and lateral bending in healthy subjects and patients with low-back disorders. *Spine*, **5**(6), 529-538.

Merriman, J.S. (1975). Stroboscopic photography as a research instrument. *Research Quarterly*, **46**, 256-261.

Miller, D.I. (1970). *A computer simulation model of the airborne phase of diving*. Unpublished doctoral dissertation, The Pennsylvania State University, University Park.

Miller, D.I., & Morrison, W.E. (1975). Prediction of segmental parameters using the Hanavan human body model. *Medicine and Science in Sports*, **7**(3), 207-212.

Miller, D.I., & Nelson, R.C. (1973). *Biomechanics of sport—A research approach* (pp. 136-138). Philadelphia: Lea and Febiger.

Miller, D.I., & Petak, K.L. (1973). Three-dimensional cinematography. In *Kinesiology III* (pp. 14-19). Washington, DC: American Alliance for Health, Physical Education, and Recreation.

Morris, J.R.W. (1973). Accelerometry—A technique for measurement of human body movements. *Journal of Biomechanics*, **6**, 729-763.

Mosely, K.D. (1974). A comparative analysis between the premotor reaction time of women athletes and women nonathletes. *Abstracts of Research Papers of American Association for Health, Physical Education, and Recreation Convention*, p. 35.

Norman, R., Sharratt, M., Pezzack, J., & Noble, E. (1976). A re-examination of the mechanical efficiency of horizontal treadmill running. In P.V. Komi (Ed.), *Biomechanics V-B* (pp. 87-93). Baltimore: University Park Press.

Norman, R.W., Bishop, P.J., Pierrynowski, M.R., & Pezzack, J.C. (1979).

Aircrew helmet protection against potential cerebral concussion in low-magnitude impacts. *Aviation Space Environmental Medicine*, **50**, 553-561.

Norman, R.W., & Komi, P.V. (1979). Electromechanical delay in skeletal muscle under normal movement conditions. *Acta Physiologica Scandinavica*, **106**, 241-248.

Normand, M.C., Lagasse, P.P., Rouillard, C.A., & Tremblay, L.E. (1982). Modifications occurring in motor programs during learning of a complex task in man. *Brain Research*, **241**(1), 87-93.

Olsen, E.A. (1956). Relationship between psychological capacities and success in college athletes. *Research Quarterly*, **27**, 78-89.

Padgaonkar, A.J., Krieger, K.W., & King, A.I. (1975). Measurement of angular acceleration of a rigid body using linear accelerometers. *Journal of Applied Mechanics*, **42**, 552-556.

Payne, A.H., Slater, W.J., & Telford, T. (1968). The use of a force platform in the study of athletic activities. A preliminary investigation. *Ergonomics*, **11**(2), 123-143.

Payton, O.D., & Kelley, D.L. (1972). Electromyographic evidence of acquisition of motor skill. *Physical Therapy*, **52**, 261-266.

Peat, M., Grahame, R.E., Fulford, R., & Quanbury, A.O. (1976). An electrogoniometer for the measurement of single plane motions. *Journal of Biomechanics*, **9**, 423-424.

Pelisse, F. (1979). The Cereval dynamic measurement force-platform. *Newsletter of the Force Platform Group, I.S.B.*, **8**, 24-34.

Person, R.S. (1958). Electromyographic investigation on coordination of activity of antagonist muscles in man during development of a motor habit. *Pavlovian Journal of Higher Nervous Activity*, **8**, 13-23.

Pezzack, J.C., Norman, R.W., & Winter, D.A. (1977). An assessment of derivative determining techniques used for motion analysis. *Journal of Biomechanics*, **10**, 377-382.

Pierson, W.R. (1956). Comparison of fencers and non fencers by psychomotor, space perception and anthropometric measures. *Research Quarterly*, **27**, 90-96.

Pierrynowski, M.R., Norman, R.W., & Winter, D.A. (1981). Mechanical energy analyses of the human during load carriage on a treadmill. *Ergonomics*, **24**(1), 1-14.

Plagenhoef, S. (1971). *Patterns of human motion. A cinematographic analysis*. Englewood Cliffs, NJ: Prentice-Hall.

Quanbury, A.O., Winter, D.A., & Reimer, G.D. (1975). Instantaneous Power and Power Flow in Body Segments During Walking. *Journal of Human Movement Studies*, **1**, 59-67.

Ralston, H.J., & Lukin, L. (1969). Energy levels in human body segments during level walking. *Ergonomics*, **12**, 39-46.

Ramey, M.R. (1973). Significance of angular momentum in long jumping. *Research Quarterly*, **44**(4), 488-497.

Ramey, M.R. (1974). The use of angular momentum in the study of long-jump take-offs. In R.C. Nelson & C.A. Morehouse (Eds.), *Biomechanics IV* (pp. 144-148). International Series on Sport Sciences, Baltimore: University Park Press.

Ramey, M.R., & Yang, A.T. (1981). A simulation procedure for human motion studies. *Journal of Biomechanics, 14*(4), 203-213.

Reid, J.G. (1967). Static strength increase and its effect upon triceps surae reflex time. *Research Quarterly, 38*, 691-697.

Robertson, G.E., & Winter, D.A. (1980). Mechanical energy generation, absorption and transfer amongst segments during walking. *Journal of Biomechanics, 13*, 845-854.

Rodrigue, D. (1981). *Validation des proprietes physiques de l'avant-bras par tomodensitometrie et par modeles geometriques.* Unpublished doctoral dissertation, Universite de Montreal, Montreal.

Schultz, A.B., & Andersson, G.B.J. (1981). Analysis of loads on the lumbar spine. *Spine, 6*(1), 76-82.

Scranton, P.E., Jr., & McMaster, J.H. (1976). Momentary distribution of forces under the foot. *Journal of Biomechanics, 9*, 45-48.

Seedhom, B.B. (1980). Mounting a force platform in a high rise building. *Newsletter of the Force Platform Group, I.S.B., 10*, 7-13.

Shapiro, R. (1978). Direct linear transformation method for three-dimensional cinematography. *Research Quarterly, 49*, 197-205.

Slater-Hammel, A.T. (1955). Comparison of reaction time measures to a visual stimulus and arm movement. *Research Quarterly, 26*, 460-479.

Smith, A.J. (1975). Photographic analysis of movement. In D.W. Grieve, D.I. Miller, D. Mitchelson, J.P. Paul, & A.J. Smith (Eds.), *Techniques for the analysis of human movement* (pp. 23-25). London: Lepus Books.

Soderberg, G.L. (1977). Below-knee amputee knee extension force-time and movement characteristics. *Physical Therapy, 58*, 966-971.

Soudan, K., & Dierskx, P. (1979). Calculations of derivatives and Fourier coefficients of human motion data, while using spline functions. *Journal of Biomechanics, 12*, 21-26.

Stepanov, A.S., & Burlakov, M.L. (1961). Electrophysiological investigation of fatigue in muscular activity. *Sechenov Physiological Journal of USSR, 47*, 43-47.

Stothart, J.P. (1973). Relationships between selected biomechanical parameters of static and dynamic muscle performance. *Medicine and Sport, 8*, 210-217.

Street, J.W. (1968). Relationship between different levels of athletic achievement and nerve conduction velocity. Unpublished master's thesis, University of Texas, Austin.

Tipton, C.M., & Karpovich, P.V. (1966). Exercise and the patella reflex. *Journal of Applied Physiology, 21*, 15-18.

Van Gheluwe, B. (1978). Computerized three-dimensional cinematography for any arbitrary camera set up. In E. Asmussen & K. Jorgensen (Eds.), *Biomechanics VI-A* (pp. 343-348). Baltimore: University Park Press.

Viitasalo, J.T., & Komi, P.V. (1981). Interrelationships between electromyographic, mechanical, muscle structure and reflex time measurements in man. *Acta Physiologica Scandinavica*, **111**, 97-103.

Vorro, J.R. (1973). Stroboscopic study of motion changes that accompany modifications and improvements in throwing performance. *Research Quarterly*, **44**, 216-226.

Vorro, J.R., & Hobart, D.J. (1974). Cinematographic analysis of intermittent modifications occurring during acquisition of novel throwing task. In R.C. Nelson & C.A. Morehouse (Eds.), *Biomechanics IV* (pp. 553-558). Baltimore: University Park Press.

Vorro, J., & Hobart, D. (1981a). Kinematic and myoelectric analysis of skill acquisition: I. 90cm subject group. *Archives of Physical Medicine and Rehabilitation*, **62**, 575-582.

Vorro, J., & Hobart, D. (1981b). Kinematic and myoelectric analysis of skill acquisition: II. 150cm subject group. *Archives of Physical Medicine and Rehabilitation*, **62**, 582-589.

Wall, J.C., Chatterji, S., & Jeffery, J.W. (1972). Human femoral cortical bone: A preliminary report on the relationship between strength and density. *Medical and Biological Engineering*, **10**, 673-676.

Wall, J.C., Chatterji, S.K., & Jeffery, J.W. (1979). Age-related changes in the density and tensile strength of human femoral cortical bone. *Calcified Tissue International*, **27**, 105-108.

Walthard, K.M., & Tchicaloff, M. (1971). Motor points. In S. Licht (Ed.), *Electrodiagnosis and Electromyography* (pp. 153-170). Baltimore: Waverly Press.

Weinbach, A.P. (1938). Contour maps, center of gravity, moment of inertia and surface area of the human body. *Human Biology*, **10**(3), 356-371.

Westerlund, J.H., & Tuttle, W.W. (1931). Relationship between running events in track and reaction time. *Research Quarterly*, **2**, 95-100.

Whitsett, C.E. (1963). *Some dynamic response characteristics of the weightless man* (AMRL-TR-63-18). Wright-Patterson Air Force Base, OH: Aerospace Medical Research Laboratories.

Wilkerson, J.D., & Cooper, J.M. (1979). Instrumentation development and validation for analyzing force applications on the balance beam. *Newsletter of the Force Platform Group, I.S.B.*, **8**, 16-23.

Willems, E.J. (1973). The relationship between the rate of tension development and the strength of a voluntary isometric muscular contraction in man. In S. Cerquiglini, A. Venerando, & J. Wartenweiler (Eds.), *Biomechanics III* (pp. 218-223). Baltimore: University Park Press.

Williams, K.R., & Cavanagh, P.R. (1983). A model for the calculation of mechanical power during distance running. *Journal of Biomechanics*, **16**(2), 115-128.

Winter, D.A. (1979a). *Biomechanics of human movement*. Toronto: John Wiley and Sons.

Winter, D.A. (1979b). A new definition of mechanical work done in human movement. *Journal of Applied Physiology*, **46**(1), 79-83.

Winter, D.A. (1980). Overall principle of lower limb support during stance phase of gait. *Journal of Biomechanics*, **13**, 923-927.

Winter, D.A., Greenlaw, R.K., & Hobson, D.A. (1972). Television computer analysis of kinematics of human gait. *Computers in Biomedical Research*, **5**, 498-504.

Winter, D.A., & Robertson, D.G.E. (1978). Joint torque and energy patterns in normal gait. *Biological Cybernetics*, **29**, 137-142.

Woltring, H.J. (1977). *Measurement and control of human movement*. Unpublished doctoral dissertation. Katholieke Universiteit, Nijmegen, The Netherlands.

Woltring, H.J. (1980). Planar control in multi-camera calibration for 3-D gain studies. *Journal of Biomechanics*, **13**, 39-48.

Wood, G.A., & Jennings, L.S. (1979). On the use of spline functions for data smoothing. *Journal of Biomechanics*, **12**, 477-479.

Woolley, C.T. (1967). *Segment masses, centers of gravity, and local moments of inertia for an analytical model of man* (LWP-228). Hampton, VA: Langley Research Center, National Aeronautics and Space Administration.

Wyss, U.P., Uozumi, T., & Polack, V.A. (1981). 3-D gait analysis using simple and inexpensive data acquisition. In *Proceedings of the 3rd Annual Conference (EMBS) (IEEE)*.

Youngen, L.A. (1969). A comparison of reaction and movement times of women athletes and non-athletes. *Research Quarterly*, **30**, 349-355.

Zatsiorsky, V., & Seluyanov, V. (1983). The mass and inertia characteristics of human body. In H. Matsui & K. Kobayaski (Eds.), *Biomechanics VIII-B* (pp. 1152-1159). Champaign, IL: Human Kinetics.

Zatiorsky, V., & Seluyanov, V. (1985). Estimation of the mass and inertia characteristics of the human body by means of the best predictive regression equations. In D. Winter, R. Norman, R. Wells, K. Hayes, & A. Patta (Eds.), *Biomechanics IX-B* (pp. 233-239). Champaign, IL: Human Kinetics.

Index

A

acceleration 10, 16-17, 30, 47, 49
accelerometer(s) 7, 16-18, 31, 56, 65, 82
action potential 60-61
angular momentum 42-44, 46, 91-92

B

ballistic 37
bone-on-bone force 3, 33, 37

C

Cartesian coordinates 44
center of gravity 10, 22, 24, 27, 42, 49, 53, 91-93, 96
center of mass 21-22, 25, 27-28, 30, 35-36, 43-45, 47
center of pressure 41
center of volume 27
cinematography 12, 33, 36, 43, 45, 74, 76, 85, 91-92
concentric 37, 84
cross-talk 88

D

damping 87
density 22, 26
digital filter 1, 81
digitizer 75
dynamics 31, 36, 43, 45, 85

E

eccentric   37, 84
efficiency   21, 31, 34, 46, 49, 51-52, 54-55, 92, 97
electrogoniometer (elgon)   1, 7, 18, 65, 82-83
electromechanical delay 62, 66-67, 70
electromyography (EMG)   7, 33, 38, 59, 62, 65-66, 68, 85, 99-100
energy   31, 46, 48-49, 50, 55-57, 94-96
ergonomics   38
Euler   43-44
external work   48, 53-55

F

fiber type   61
finite element   27, 29
force platform (plate)   7, 36, 39-40, 49, 56, 85, 88-89, 91-92, 100
Fourier   1, 81
free-body diagram   36
frequency response   17, 87

G

gamma-scanner   27
ground reaction force   33, 35-36, 39, 45, 73, 84

H

hydrostatic   27
hysteresis   87-88, 90

I

impact   32
impulse   32, 34-35, 42, 46, 91
inertia   22, 38, 83
internal work   48, 53-54
ISEK   99
isometric   38, 53

J

joint reaction force   33-37, 45, 84-85

K

kinematic(s)   7, 9, 11-13, 20, 24, 31, 45, 83, 92, 97
kinetic energy   46, 56-57, 93-94
kinetics   7, 11, 21, 31, 34, 45

L

latency   61, 65
light emitting diode (LED)   41
linear programming   38, 85
linearity   87-88, 90
linked-segment model   36

M

mass   21, 22, 24, 30, 36, 45, 47
moment of inertia   22-23, 27-30, 32, 34, 36, 43, 47, 84, 91, 96
momentum   32, 34-35, 42, 91
motor task   60
motor time   60, 61, 65-67
motor unit   62
muscular force   33-36
muscular torque   33, 84

N

natural frequency   41, 89-90

O

optimization   37, 85
optoelectric   14, 78-79

P

parallel axis theorem   23
potential energy   46, 56-57, 93-94
potentiometer   7, 82-83
power   2, 31, 45, 98
premotor time   60-61, 65-66
pressure   33, 35, 42, 45

Q

quick-release method   29-30

R

radius of gyration   23, 27
reaction change   25, 27
reaction time   60, 63, 66
reflex(es)   61, 63, 69
resonance   88
rigid body   43

S

sampling rate   80-81
sampling theorem   81
Selspot   14, 78, 96
sensitivity   87, 90
Simpson's Rule   92
smoothing   81, 85
spline functions   81
statics   36
stroboscopy   13, 77-78

T

television (TV)   15, 79-80
torque   24, 32, 39-40, 47-49
trapezoidal rule   92

V

Varignon's Theorem   22, 28
volume   21, 26, 28

W

Watsmart   15, 79
weight   21, 22, 47
work   31, 46-50, 52-57, 94, 96